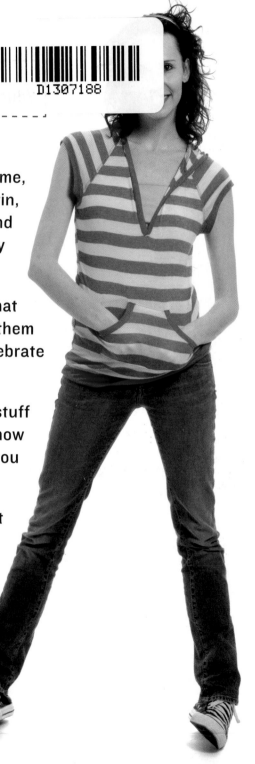

# bod·y dra·ma \BOD-ee DRAH

*noun*

① Physical issues that mortify, shame, humiliate, disconcert, abash, chagrin, fluster, distress, embarrass, and threaten to ruin your life . . . directly in front of your crush.

② Things you feel so helpless about that you write to Santa asking him to fix them for Christmas, even if you don't celebrate the holiday.

③ Stinky, strange, scary, stressful stuff you don't even want your pets to know about, let alone your parents . . . so you pretend that it doesn't exist.

④ That which you're paranoid about ending up on the bathroom wall, or worse, someone's MySpace page.

⑤ What this book's all about.

# BODY

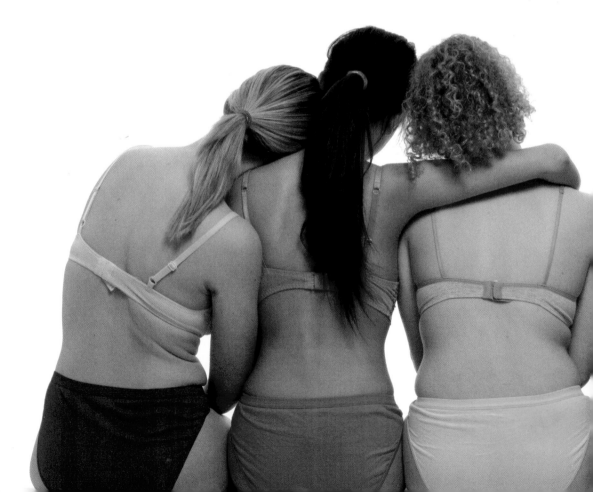

# DRAMA

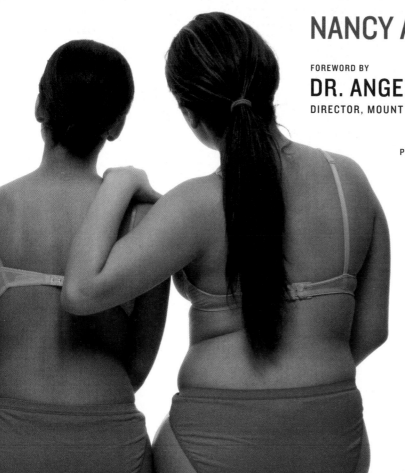

NANCY AMANDA REDD

FOREWORD BY
## DR. ANGELA DIAZ
DIRECTOR, MOUNT SINAI ADOLESCENT HEALTH CENTER

PHOTOGRAPHY BY **KELLY KLINE**

GOTHAM BOOKS

GOTHAM BOOKS
Published by Penguin Group (USA) Inc.
375 Hudson Street, New York, New York 10014, U.S.A.

Penguin Group (Canada), 90 Eglinton Avenue East, Suite
700, Toronto, Ontario M4P 2Y3, Canada (a division of
Pearson Penguin Canada Inc.); Penguin Books Ltd, 80
Strand, London WC2R 0RL, England; Penguin Ireland,
25 St Stephen's Green, Dublin 2, Ireland (a division of
Penguin Books Ltd); Penguin Group (Australia), 250
Camberwell Road, Camberwell, Victoria 3124, Australia
(a division of Pearson Australia Group Pty Ltd); Penguin
Books India Pvt Ltd, 11 Community Centre, Panchsheel
Park, New Delhi – 110 017, India; Penguin Group (NZ), 67
Apollo Drive, Rosedale, North Shore 0632, New Zealand
(a division of Pearson New Zealand Ltd); Penguin Books
(South Africa) (Pty) Ltd, 24 Sturdee Avenue, Rosebank,
Johannesburg 2196, South Africa

Penguin Books Ltd, Registered Offices:
80 Strand, London WC2R 0RL, England

Published by Gotham Books, a member of Penguin Group
(USA) Inc.

Gotham Books and the skyscraper logo are trademarks of
Penguin Group (USA) Inc.

Library of Congress Cataloging-in-Publication Data has been
applied for.

First printing, January 2008
10  9  8  7  6  5  4  3  2  1

ISBN 978-1-592-40326-4
Printed in the United States of America

Produced in association with Herter Studio LLC
www.herterstudio.com

While the author has made every effort to provide accurate
telephone numbers and Internet addresses at the time of
publication, neither the publisher nor the author assumes
any responsibility for errors, or for changes that occur after
publication. Further, the publisher does not have any control
over and does not assume any responsibility for author or
third-party Web sites or their content.

PUBLISHER'S NOTE: Neither the publisher nor the author is
engaged in rendering professional advice or services to the
individual reader. The ideas, procedures, and suggestions
contained in this book are not intended as a substitute for
consulting with your physician. All matters regarding your
health require medical supervision. Neither the author nor
the publisher shall be liable or responsible for any loss or
damage allegedly arising from any information or suggestion
in this book.

*To Rupak,*
*for being the first to encourage me to write this book,*
*for knowing me better than I know myself,*
*and for loving me just as I am*

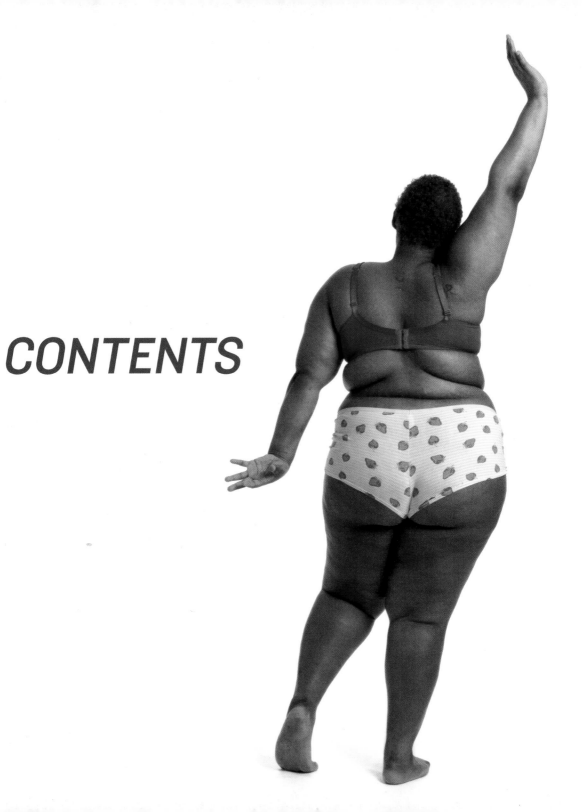

# CONTENTS

# SKIN

# BOOBS

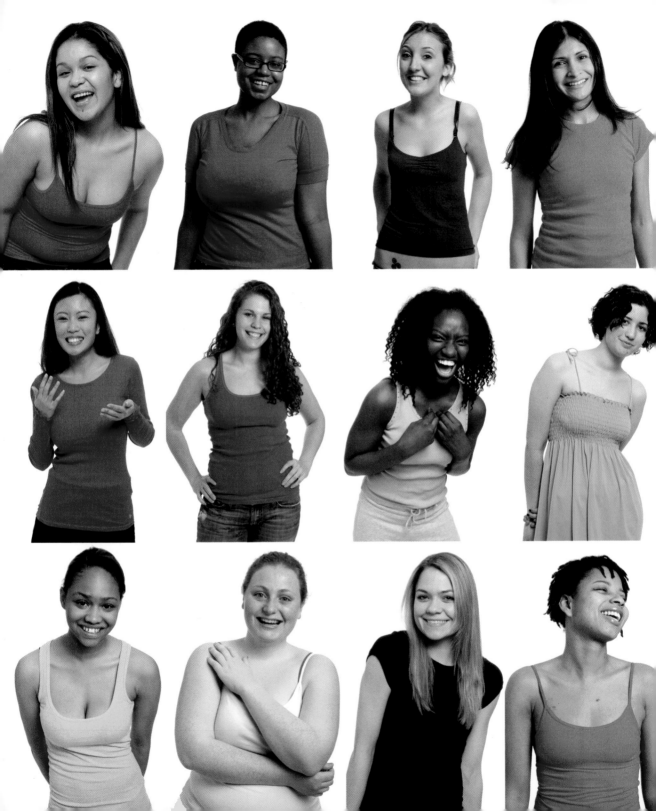

# THE MANY FACES OF
# NORMAL

## BY DR. ANGELA DIAZ
### Director of the Mount Sinai Adolescent Health Center, New York City

During my twenty-five years as a doctor specializing in adolescent medicine and as director of the Mount Sinai Adolescent Health Center in New York City, which serves 10,000 teens every year and is the largest and most comprehensive adolescent health center in the United States, I have seen, diagnosed, and treated thousands of young women dealing with every drama discussed in this book—from breast size to sexually transmitted infections.

As initially shocking or graphic as its contents may seem, *Body Drama* reflects the concerns I deal with daily. It is frequently necessary to spend time allaying the fears of female adolescent patients, explaining that there isn't one type of "normal" and that vaginas, breasts, and other body parts come in all shapes and sizes. Still, reassurance is often not enough, and more than a verbal OK is needed. As the saying goes, "One picture is worth a thousand words."

More than ever, today's girls need role models—and not just in school. They need body role models. My patients, like the young women featured in this book, have some of the most beautiful, healthy physiques around, but none of them look like the women they see in fashion magazines or on television. Today's young women need real images—not misleading illustrations and medical jargon. They need reality checks and reassurance. They need this book.

By proudly presenting what real women actually look like and what women's bodies naturally go through, *Body Drama* takes a major stride toward eradicating the dislike and embarrassment that women have learned to feel about their bodies. Because of shame and ignorance, the doctor's office is too frequently a teen's last resort. Many young women come to my center with fears, concerns, and health issues that have plagued them for a long time. When they need treatment, their situations have often worsened because of this delay. Very often they are healthy but in need of information or counsel. Too often they feel bad about themselves, and their unfounded fears could have been allayed. When asked why they waited so long to get help, the answers include "I was embarrassed" or "I didn't know it was that big a deal" or "I thought it was hopeless." Many teens say, "There is nowhere to go."

So, instead of seeking professional help, young women turn to more comfortable sources, such as friends or the anonymous Internet, leading to an abundance of misinformation being shared. At times, teenage circles offer shockingly erroneous advice that confounds even a basic comprehension of simple body facts. Are boys right when they say that darker labia are caused by an internal illness? Are blood clots during menstruation really a sign of cancer? Is Coca-Cola an effective spermicide? All of these are myths easily disproved at the doctor's office, but because some girls are too afraid (or don't know how) to seek help face-to-face, and because they don't understand the medical terminology that credible sources use, they too often turn to more easily digestible, but misleading, chat rooms and gossip instead of to a professional who has the knowledge and ability to help them.

Because of Nancy Redd's youth and her extensive work with teenagers, she knows what matters most to young women, and her readers will relate to, enjoy, and find comfort in her fresh, intelligent, and powerful voice. *Body Drama* presents reliable information in a "medical textbook meets *Seventeen* magazine" way. Best of all, this groundbreaking book not only talks about the many faces of normal, but it also shows those faces via unaltered photos of real young women, accompanied by solid advice written in a language young women can understand.

*Body Drama* enables the reader to take a more robust, wholesome, and candid approach to deciding which body dramas are medical crises and which are not. *Body Drama* tells readers when and how to seek medical help and what to expect from professional care. Such crucial information is often omitted from advice texts or presented in language that is too technical to be understood easily.

This book will help health providers, parents, and others who deal with fearful, stressed-out teen girls. *Body Drama* is a unique, unprecedented book that will open a treasure chest of questions and answers for the young woman reader (and her parents). It will help eradicate much ignorance and many misconceptions about real women's bodies.

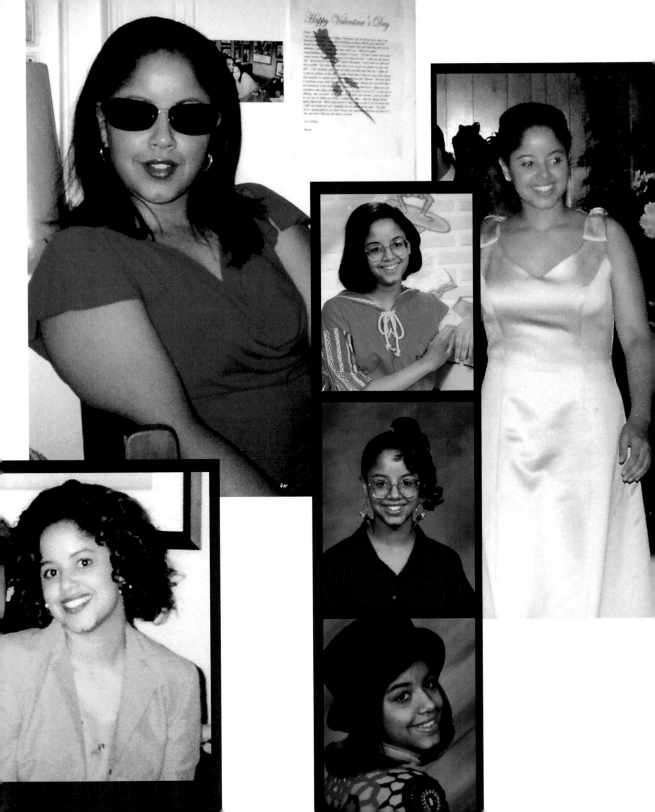

# NO BODY'S
# PERFECT

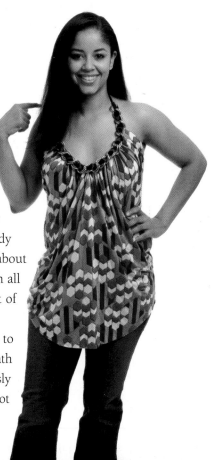

You'd think a Miss America swimsuit winner would feel completely confident about her body, right? Think again! What? You feel like you're the first girl in the world to suffer from back acne, saggy breasts, or bad breath? Puh-leaze! I've been dealing with body drama almost since the day I was born. *So have I,* you might be thinking, but the problem is that I, like a lot of you, thought I was the only one who felt that her body was a natural disaster. For the longest time, I hated my body and all the stuff it did (and didn't) do. Although I was happy about how I looked in nice outfits and perfect makeup, underneath all the layers I truly thought I was a weird, stinky girl with a lot of body problems.

I don't know about you, but I've *always* been curious to know what other women's bodies *really* look like underneath their clothes. Not sexually, but in a "is my body as hideously deformed as I think it is?" kind of way. Lacking a sister (and not having the infamous "locker room experience" in high school), I had no way of knowing if the gross stuff that happened to me was normal. Was I the only one who grew hair in strange places? Found yucky stuff in my underwear? Had deep dents on my thighs? Did other women have clots during their period or poo problems or pimples on their backs? From what I saw in the media, it certainly didn't seem that they did. No one on TV or in magazines ever had pit stains or stretch marks! Unfortunately, aside from airbrushed pornography and too-thin supermodels, the unrealistic illustrations that all other body books use to show "normal" women were the only bodies I could sneak peeks at.

I couldn't find real photographs of actual women, and I couldn't find the help I needed on other embarrassing issues. Because legitimate guidance on how to deal with day-to-day worries like bad breath, embarrassing nipple hair, ashy skin, or split ends didn't exist, I assumed I was the only one who was doomed to suffer from them.

We girls are under tremendous pressure to conform to absurd physical ideals, but we have too few worthwhile tools to help us understand ourselves and care for our natural bodily leaks, creaks, and crevices. It's just not fair! Let's face it: Most health books are filled with bland information and boring, barely accurate drawings. I haven't a clue who the model was for the drawing of the naked woman in the body book I got for my thirteenth birthday, but she in no way resembled ME. When comparing and contrasting my body parts to the vaguely sketched ones in health books, I felt like the punch line of a cruel joke. And don't get me started on the penciled pictures detailing how to give myself a breast exam! The crudely drawn charcoal boob looked nothing like my own! How can we expect cartoons to teach us how to take care of ourselves and convince us that our bodies are normal and OK?

Our educational system spends millions of dollars creating detailed health programs, but those programs skip over the ABCs of basic body smarts. We've been so focused (and understandably so) on *sexual* education that we have completely ignored *body* education. By the end of eighth grade, I'd been through three mandatory, week-long rounds of sex ed, and I could easily spout off facts about how syphilis was a curable STI but HIV was not, and why the "pull-out" method isn't an effective way to avoid pregnancy. Still, for all my knowledge on how to keep bad things from happening to my body in the *future,* I had NO idea how to deal with the body issues I faced every day. Sure, it was nice to know that you can't get HIV from kissing, but fourteen-year-old me was too busy worrying about my dandruff to even consider kissing someone, let alone having sex! All I wanted was solutions to the simple, yet traumatic, issues I was dealing with daily. And I know now that I'm not the only one. C'mon . . . how can we respect and protect our bodies if we don't know what real bodies look like? If we can hardly utter the word *vagina,* much less peek at it without feeling dirty, how can we own and love it and ourselves?

Enter *Body Drama,* the book I wish I'd had as a teen and the book that all young women need today more than ever before. When I first planned this project, many people thought I was crazy. With wrinkled noses, they'd say, "Who wants to see pictures of belly rolls and floppy boobs?" or "Talking about this stuff is disgusting!" One friend even begged me to use a fake name, saying that my Harvard honors degree and my "outstanding reputation" would be down the toilet. After all, who wants to be affiliated with poo problems?

Actually, *I* do! We deserve to celebrate, not hide, our differences and uniqueness by seeing our real selves in print! Why should we be forced to ignore natural bodily functions or to feel ashamed of them? Young women shouldn't be left searching blindly for solutions to their body dramas—especially considering that much of the information "out there" is inaccurate, perhaps even dangerous. From discharge to dry skin, from vaginal smells to STIs, *Body Drama* closes the current gap in women's health education by going beyond our periods and providing practical and entertaining information, photographs, and anecdotes that describe how real bodies look and how they function—the good, the bad, as well as the ugly, the funky, and the admittedly gross.

As you'll see from the embarrassing personal experiences that I've shared in this book, I'm an expert on body dramas, but I'm no medical professional. To obtain the best information possible, I called on Dr. Angela Diaz, director of America's most prestigious medical clinic for teens at the Mount Sinai Adolescent Health Center in New York City. She and her staff see over 10,000 teenagers a year, many of whom come to the clinic with the same body dramas that are discussed in this book. She helped me select the best information and advice to share, and brought her invaluable firsthand experience to the project as well.

So just what does *Body Drama* cover? If you're still reading this introduction and haven't already eagerly flipped to the "shape spread" (my favorite part of the book, pages 246–247), let me explain. There are five distinct parts: skin, boobs, "down there," hair/mouth/nails, and shape. The issues discussed in each part are described as "dramas," since that's how they make us feel when they happen. It may seem like the end of your world if you fry your hair with a flat iron, or you might think that you'll never find love because your vagina smells, but as you'll see in this book, there is a light at the end of the tunnel.

*Body Drama* covers the topics we've all fretted about (whether we admit it or not) but never had the right resource to turn to. I've talked with hundreds of girls and

I know from personal experience what issues keep you up at night, what topics you want to learn about, what information you need when dealing with dramas, and where you can go to get help when you need it. Guaranteed, after reading this, you'll know what real bodies in every shape, size, and ethnicity look like. You will also see how many variations of "normal" women exist, and you'll know how to take good care of your own special body. From a flat butt to flatulence to a third nipple to a triple-A-cup chest—these words describe body parts and issues we all deal with, but they don't make us who we are. How we choose to work with what we have does. This book is designed to help you realize—and rejoice!—that every body is different. No matter what size or shape you are, you deal with body drama, and you are not alone!

*Nancy Redd, January 2008*

# BODY

# DRAMA

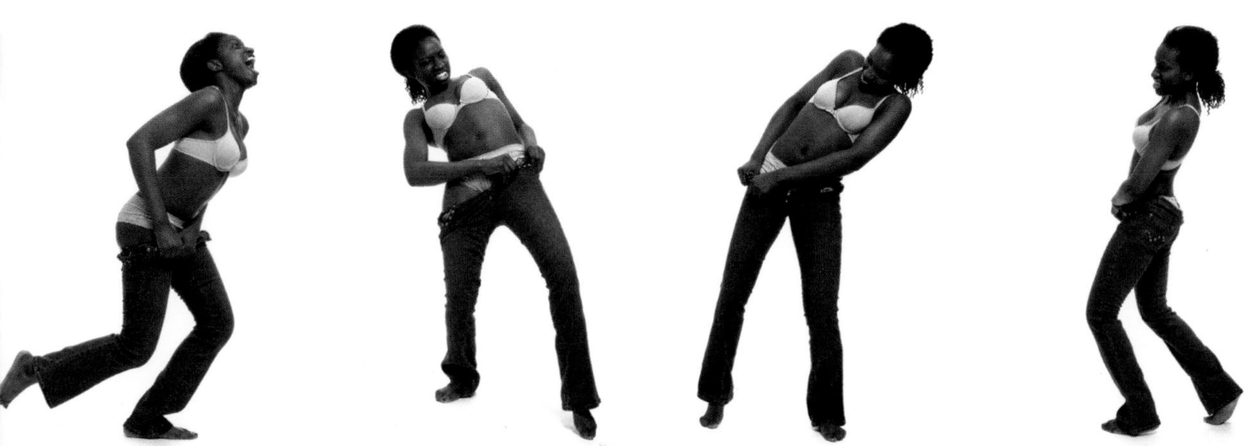

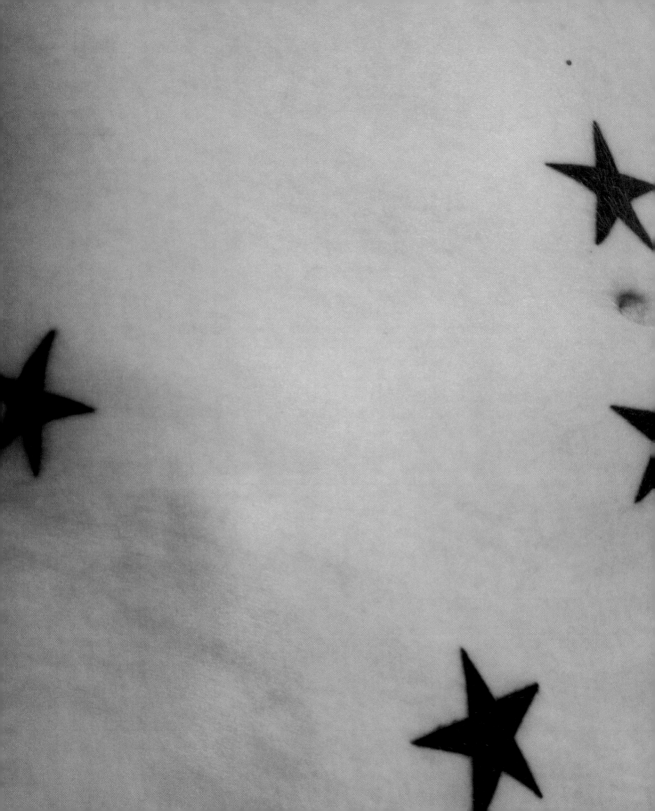

# SKIN

Dealing with my skin was once rougher than an unsoaked foot callus. Pimples, dandruff, ashy skin, and stinky sweat threatened to take over my life, and although I tried every deodorant I could find and drank enough water to pee an ocean, nothing seemed to work. The lightest workout in gym class left me completely drenched and reeking while my fresh-smelling friends remained dry as deserts . . . leading me to conveniently fall "sick" during that forty-five-minute class as often as possible.

I was stuck with bumpy, funky skin for years, but it turns out I wasn't alone. Looking back at my yearbooks, I see no sweat stains under my armpits, and my pimples look no worse than my classmates'. But at the time, it seemed that none of my friends' skin caused them as much trouble as mine caused me. I had no idea that every girl feels that way about her own issues—as if her problems are the worst in the world.

By senior year, my body started getting it together. My face was smoother and I didn't seem to smell as bad. Had drinking all of that water really helped? Was it my deodorant and perfectly concealing make-up? Or had my hormones decided to calm down and cut me some slack?

Honestly, I never thought about it. I was just glad that the bumps were behind me—and no longer on my behind!

Our skin puts us through a lot of trauma, but we're not too easy on it either. From makeup left on overnight, to razor burn from a dull blade, to dehydration in a super-hot shower, to pain from a strangely placed piercing, our skin survives a lot of self-inflicted damage. No one has ever died from a prominent pimple or stinky sweat, but skin issues sure can kill self-esteem. Luckily, this chapter is here to help you banish breakouts and obliterate odors without breaking a sweat!

# My face is a zit factory.

## WHAT'S GOING ON?

Does it seem as if your face has more craters than the moon, while it's smooth sailing for everyone else's skin? The medical term for blackheads, whiteheads, and other pimples you find on your face and body is *acne,* and it's actually classified by some as a disease (yes, disease!) of the oil glands.

Oil glands, also medically known as sebaceous **(sih-BAY-shus)** glands, are found in our hair follicles, which cover our entire body. When a follicle clogs up with oil, dirt, or bacteria, zits appear. Since follicles are found everywhere except on the palms of your hands and the soles of your feet, it's also possible to get pimples anywhere on your body, including your face, neck, arms, back, butt, legs, and breasts. (Find out how to deal with "bacne" on page 34.)

*A number of things affect acne:*
- Excessive sebum (oil) blocking your follicles and pores (the evil base of nearly all pimples);
- Emotional stress (which causes you to produce more pore-blocking sebum);
- Dead skin cells and bacteria mixing with sebum, infecting your follicles and pores (a nasty combination);
- Voodoo curses (OK, that's not possible, although it might seem like a hex when that day-of-the-prom pimple pops up).

Acne is especially terrible between the ages of fourteen and nineteen, when our bodies start revving their oil engines, inevitably causing clogs and producing a mind-boggling number of pimples, especially on our faces. What's more, genes may also be responsible for PFS (Pizza-Face Syndrome). If your parents didn't have many zits as teens, chances are you're in the clear, too. But if you notice that they've torn all their photos out of their yearbooks, get ready to combat your skin.

## HOW DO I DEAL?

Are your oil-wells-for-pores drilling your self-esteem into the ground? Be patient. Acne usually improves in your late teens or early twenties as your body's oil production slows down. If you can't wait for nature to take its course, here are some helpful tips:

**Don't pop.** Squeezing a zit might make you feel proactive, but you're working against yourself. You'll never be able to empty all the pus from the pore, and you could end up leaving a permanent scar. You are also inviting infections.

**Stay clean.** Cleansing helps remove the oil, sweat, dead skin cells, and bacteria that infect your pores and follicles. Wash your face with a gentle cleanser (perhaps one with acne-fighting ingredients, such as benzoyl peroxide or salicylic acid) in the morning, at night, and after working out. Don't go too scrub crazy, though: Using rough exfoliants and scrubbing until you're red in the face irritates your skin and can worsen the problem. For best results, use your fingertips to softly massage the cleanser into your face, rinse well, and pat your skin dry afterward. To keep your face fresh throughout the day, consider carrying around a travel-size cleanser to use during a midday break.

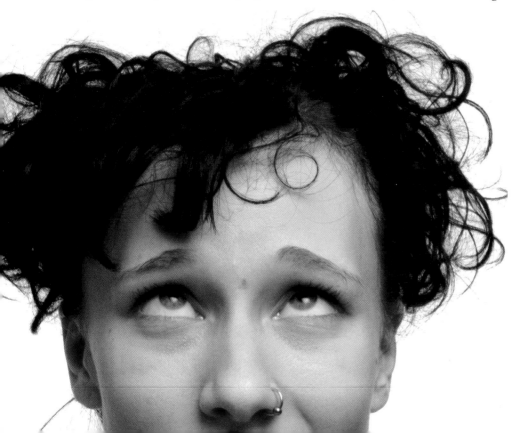

Or, oil-absorbing blotting sheets (available at any drugstore) are an inexpensive and easy-to-use option to soak up excess oils.

**Check your products.** If you're using hair oil, gel, or spray that might be dripping onto your forehead or cheeks, the product could easily be the cause of your pimples. Also, switch your washcloth or rinse your facial brush in hot water after every use, because either one can harbor acne-aggravating bacteria.

**Hats off.** If you often wear a helmet, hat, or headband and you're noticing a bunch of brow bumps, the constant friction of sweaty, dirty, bacteria-covered material against your forehead is a likely culprit.

**Chill out.** It's easy to freak out about your skin, but the more you stress, the worse your skin gets. Try exercising for stress relief, but suds up afterward! Sweat on your skin promotes bacterial growth that could lead to a fresh crop of zits.

**Patience.** While zits can show up overnight, they often take weeks to calm down after a flare-up. While you wait, be sure to get enough sleep, and drink at least eight glasses of water daily to help your skin heal.

If over-the-counter cleansers and tweaks in your skin care routine don't seem to make a difference, *see your doctor.* He or she can give you some solid medical advice and perhaps prescribe medication to help clear your skin.

## WHAT IF THEY NOTICE?

Most people find themselves playing connect the dots on their face at some point (especially during puberty), so rest assured that you aren't the only one dealing with pimples. While you might be stuck with spots this week, when you're in the clear next month, the spots might have migrated onto your big crush! Men get worse acne than women do, so in that regard we're pretty lucky! Don't shy away from society because of your skin. Just take care of yourself (turn to page 32 to learn how to give yourself a facial) and don't make a big deal about the bumps you have. Absolutely everyone breaks out, and the zits you notice most are your own!

# TYPES OF PIMPLES

Know your enemies! Blocked pores can lead to a variety of breakouts. With this list, you'll know exactly what you're dealing with when you spy a skin spot.

Papules, pustules, nodules, and cysts are the more severe forms of acne. If they're cropping up on your cheek, *see a doctor* for treatment and medication to reduce the spots and to minimize scarring.

### In Order of Severity (Least to Worst)

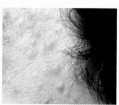

### WHITEHEADS

*Hair follicles blocked with oil, bacteria, and dead cells appear to have white "heads." Because these pimples stay underneath the surface of the skin, they clear up faster than other types.*

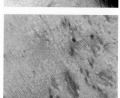

### BLACKHEADS

*Blocked hair follicles that rise to the surface of the skin. They're not black because of dirt. The oil inside turns darker once it mixes with the oxygen in the air.*

### PAPULES AND PUSTULES

*Papules are inflamed, small bumps that are tender to the touch. Pustules are larger, redder bumps that have white, pus-filled "heads."*

### NODULES

*Hard and painful red bumps that are embedded deeply in the skin and can last for months, causing scarring.*

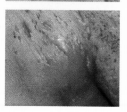

### CYSTS

*Huge, nodulelike red bumps that are filled with pus. They are often very painful. They can become infected and inflamed, and they can cause extreme scarring.*

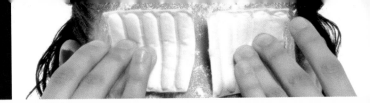

Treat yourself to a facial with stuff you've already got in your house! Aspirin isn't just for headaches. A form of salicylic acid—a proven pimple reducer—is an ingredient in aspirin, and in crushed form, aspirin can exfoliate your skin. Kick back with this mask once or twice a month and you'll get brighter skin and relieve some stress in the process.

☀ **CAUTION:** If you're allergic to aspirin when you take it orally, do not use this mask. Instead, turn to page 59 for a different facial treatment.

### WHAT YOU NEED:

3 washcloths or hand towels • your usual face cleanser • 6 adult-size aspirin tablets • I metal spoon • I plate • water • chilled toner or astringent (Stick your usual bottle in the fridge for a couple of hours.) • chilled moisturizer (Put your regular moisturizer in the fridge, too.) • 2 cotton pads

### WHAT TO DO:

① Wash your face with your regular cleanser and pat dry.

② Using the back of your spoon, crush the aspirin tablets on a plate. Add a few drops of water, mixing well and adding more until you have a thick paste. If you add too much water, don't worry. It will evaporate.

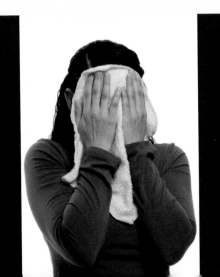

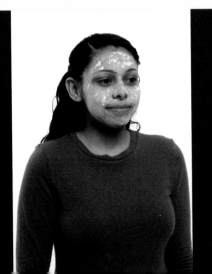

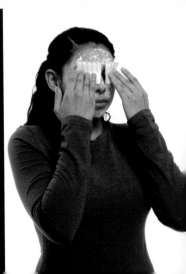

③ Rinse a washcloth in warm, nearly hot water and wring out the moisture.

④ Cover your face with the washcloth, keeping it there until it is almost cold.

⑤ Remove the washcloth and test the aspirin paste. If it's dried out a bit, add some more water until it is spreadable.

⑥ Avoiding your eyes, use your fingertips to spread the paste all over your face, making sure to get it on the sides of your nose.

⑦ Dampen two cotton pads with warm water and cover your eyes for a few minutes. You may want to lie down and relax during this step!

⑧ Wait until the mask dries and is crumbly to the touch. Wet another washcloth in warm, nearly hot water.

⑨ Cover your face with the washcloth, pressing down with your fingertips to help remove the mask. Let the washcloth sit until it's almost cold. Then use it to wipe away the rest of the mask, rewetting if necessary.

⑩ Apply the chilled toner or astringent all over your face, followed by the chilled moisturizer, massaging your skin with slow, soothing strokes, especially around your temples and neck.

Voila! Great skin for pennies!

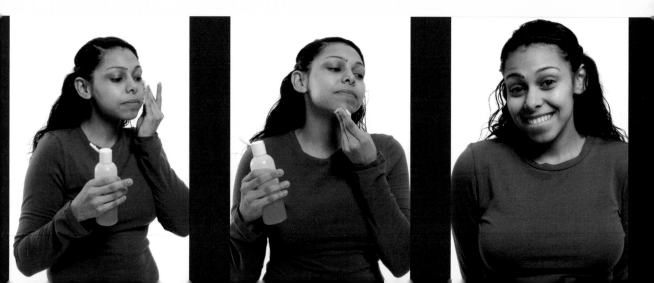

# I have acne on my butt and back.

## WHAT'S GOING ON?

Pimples on your face are problems enough, but unsightly "bacne" and "buttne" (acne that shows up on your butt and back) can be the bane of your existence. Bacne comes in all forms of pimples and is a literal pain in the butt. The same substance that causes facial acne—sebum (oil) mixing with bacteria and sweat that infects and clogs your follicles—also leads to butt and back bumps. Unlike pimples on your face, pimples where the sun doesn't shine are constantly coming in contact with the clothes that cover them, and the friction from the fabric does *not* feel good.

## HOW DO I DEAL?

To maintain a beautiful back and butt, follow these simple steps:

**Loosen up.** Tight clothing traps dirt and perspiration, creating the perfect breeding ground for bacne-causing bacteria. As soon as you get back from a workout, peel off those stinky sweats. If at all possible, stick with cotton fabrics that allow your body to breathe. Moisture-trapping spandex tempts bacteria to multiply faster, which can make your bacne worse.

**Stay clean.** Shower immediately after getting dirty or exercising. The less time oil and bacteria spend on your skin, the harder it will be for them to infiltrate your pores.

**Guzzle water** often to keep your body's waste removal processes functioning at top efficiency.

**Treat the worst spots** with the acne medicine or astringent you use on your face, but ONLY if the pimples are nowhere near your genitals.

Have past bouts with bacne left you with dark spots and scars? The answer is probably yes, but don't worry. Things will improve over time. As your skin renews and rejuvenates, most of your skin stains will disappear.

## WHAT IF THEY NOTICE?

Worried that people are laughing behind your back, about your back? Don't be—others probably haven't even noticed! You've probably got your problem covered most of the time, except when you wear something strapless or with a V-neck. Then, body makeup or a fabulous shawl can help you keep your bacne under wraps!

"Bacne"                          "Buttne"

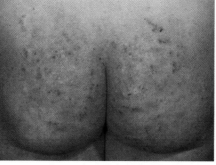

While we're busy trying to cover our scars, some cultures consider them so beautiful they create them on purpose! Many African tribes practice a ritual called scarification, where a skilled carver cuts village women and men hundreds of times all over their bodies in intricate patterns. Then, salt is rubbed into the wounds, irritating them. The irritation causes the resulting scar tissue to be raised. Once healed, textured works of art permanently decorate the person's back, breasts, stomach, forehead, and cheeks. Often, these scars are a sign of maturity and social class; unscarred skin is considered much less attractive.

# OTHER TYPES OF BODY BUMPS

From the bottoms of our feet to the tips of our noses, pimples aren't the only kinds of bumps our bodies are prone to.

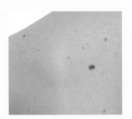

### MOLES

*Clusters of pigmented cells that are hereditary, can sprout hair, and should be checked frequently because some of them can become cancerous (see page 45 for more information).*

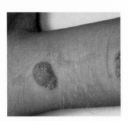

### WARTS

*Rough-surfaced, cauliflowerlike bumps that are caused by a strain of human papilloma virus (HPV—see page 123 for more information). Nearly two-thirds of all warts disappear on their own within two years, but they can also be treated or removed by a doctor or with over-the-counter medication.*

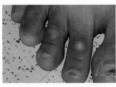

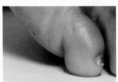

### CALLUSES AND CORNS

*Areas of toughened skin on feet and hands formed by excess pressure, such as running, strumming the guitar, or performing manual labor. Calluses are painless, hardened bumps of skin that form on toes and fingers, the soles of feet, and the palms of hands. Corns are similar to calluses in appearance but actually have internal cores with sharp points on the bottom that press into the skin, causing pain. Corns usually appear on the tops or sides of toes. Corns and calluses are annoying but not harmful. Both can sometimes be removed by buffing them away yourself with a pumice stone, with over-the-counter medicine, or by having your doctor do it. Corns and calluses on the feet can be prevented with corrective shoe inserts, while hand calluses can be prevented with gloves.*

# COLD SORE, HERPES, OR BOTH?

Does it look as if someone put out a cigarette on your upper lip? Don't think that you're doomed forever. It's estimated that nine out of ten people will be exposed to herpes at some point in their lives. There are many strands of herpes, some of which are not sexually transmitted infections (STIs) but that still cause cold sores.

While genital sores that reappear throughout one's life are usually caused by the herpes simplex virus type 2 (HSV-2), the short-lived mouth sores known as fever blisters or cold sores are typically caused by the herpes simplex virus type I (HSV-I).

All types of herpes are contagious, especially during an outbreak, so be responsible: Avoid smooching and sharing utensils with others until all signs of the sore have vanished. If a cold sore sprouts on you or your partner, do not give or receive oral sex. Why? Because the types of herpes don't always stay where they belong!

Although technically HSV-I is not a sexually transmitted infection, more and more young adults are catching it in their genital area after receiving oral sex from someone who has a cold sore. And, if you perform oral sex on someone with genital herpes, the virus can infect your mouth!

It isn't hard to miss an outbreak, but since HSV-2 and HSV-I can look identical, determining the difference is not simple and is best left to a doctor. So, if you're sexually active (oral sex counts), and an eruption appears, DON'T try to diagnose yourself. *See your doctor* while the spot is still visible, as it's much harder to detect herpes when there's not an outbreak. Even if it's just a cold sore, your doctor may provide you with a prescription to help you heal faster.

For more information on sexually transmitted herpes, see page 122.

# I sweat more than other girls do.

## WHAT'S GOING ON?

Everybody sweats, but genes predispose some of us to sweat more than others (thanks, Grandma). When working out or sitting in the hot sun, it's hard to tell a person who sweats excessively apart from everyone else because we all perspire to help keep our body's temperature at a normal level. But for those with trigger-happy sweat glands, stress alone can get the perspiration flowing, even while sitting in a cool breeze. Stress-induced pit stains, forehead beads, and slick palms can be noticeable and embarrassing, and stressing about stress sweat only leads to more . . . sweating! Will the cycle ever end? ARRGH!

Are you sweating bullets just reading this? Do you change your shirt a couple of times on a normal day because of sweat? Does your sweat often soak through a few layers? Have you thrown away pit-stained clothes? If so, you have loads of company: Nearly eight million Americans say they deal with hyperhidrosis **(hie-per-hie-DROH-sis)**, the medical term for excessive sweating.

## HOW DO I DEAL?

Aspiring to less frequent perspiring? First things first: Just because you sweat doesn't mean you have to stink. Avoid strong-smelling or spicy foods such as onions and garlic because their odors can linger in your skin, seeping out when you sweat.

Your clothing fabric might be fueling your underarm fire. For example, polyester, rayon, and silk are not breathable fabrics, so once your body starts heating up, these materials just trap the warmth. Exchange your stifling shirts for ones made of cotton, which is always the most comfortable, breathable fabric.

Check to see if your current deodorant has the word *antiperspirant* on the label. If it doesn't, your deodorant may be masking the funk without preventing the flow. Antiperspirants come in many forms, so explore different sticks, sprays, creams, and powders until you find one that works well. Finding your feet to be part of the problem? Keep them as dry as possible, changing socks often. There are also over-the-counter products and prescriptions sold specifically for sweaty toes.

These and many more options are available at any drugstore, and you can always ask the pharmacist for a recommendation if you feel overwhelmed.

If after experimenting you find that an over-the-counter antiperspirant doesn't work wonders on your wetness, *see your doctor.* There are prescription options available that can be quite effective for sweaty palms and axillary (underarm) hyperhidrosis.

If you still feel that none of these methods is stopping your sweat, there are a few more extreme options (with considerable side effects), such as mild electrical shocks called iontophoresis **(eye-on-tuh-fuh-REE-sis)**, botox injections, and even surgery. These more intense treatment methods can take a toll on your body in other ways, but they're worth considering if you're in a really, really sticky situation. Sometimes, excessive sweating is a symptom of another medical condition, such as an anxiety disorder, so if you're concerned about the amount you're perspiring, or if you're interested in some stronger sweat-reducing solutions, checking in with your doctor is a slick move.

## WHAT IF THEY NOTICE?

If you feel less hot because of your body's intense efforts to cool itself at inopportune times, there are some things you can do to keep sweat from ruining your social climate.

A few cosmetic lines offer oil-absorbing blotting sheets to help you save face, or you might keep a handkerchief handy for soaking up those telltale brow beads.

Predict a pit problem? You can protect your outfit (and your dignity) by layering your clothing with a short-sleeved cotton undershirt (or two). Also, special armpit pads can be worn to keep extra moisture under wraps. To be prepared for the next sunny day that makes your pits rain, consider stashing fresh shirts and a jacket in your car or locker to have on sweat standby.

I bathe every day but I still smell.

## WHAT'S GOING ON?

If you've recently been feeling funky for reasons other than your great fashion style, your "stink" glands—known medically as the apocrine **(AP-uh-krin)** glands—have probably become more active. Most of your body is covered in sweat glands, but apocrine glands are the ones situated in areas such as your genitals and underarms. Besides their location, what makes apocrine glands unique is that the sweat they secrete is laced with fat and protein. Body odor is created when this nutrient-rich sweat mixes with the bacteria and dirt that are trapped by your skin and body hair over the course of a normal day.

*fast fact*

*NEWSFLASH! Deodorants with antiperspirants don't cause cancer! For years, people thought that the aluminum in some sweat-stopping deodorants might block pores, causing cancer, but recent studies have found no such link.*

## HOW DO I DEAL?

Staying stink-free can be challenging. There are many components to how we smell, our skin being only one of them. Many times, it's not our body, but our clothes, that reek. Wearing the same outfits without washing them first can lead to odor problems. Even items like jackets and jeans need to be cleaned fairly often. If they don't pass the sniff test, neither will you.

Also, how's your diet? Even if you're squeaky clean, certain foods can ooze odor from your pores, and the smell of your breath might not be helping your overall aroma, either.

Finally, of course you know to keep your body clean, but bathing *often* is not as important as bathing *properly*. To get truly clean, get into every one of your body's nooks and crannies with soap and water. Any spot that grows hair also grows bad-smelling bacteria, so leave no spot unwashed.

*Here's a cheat sheet for the tub or shower:*

- Using soap or body wash, suds up a clean washcloth, shower mitt, or loofah and get ready to start working head-to-toe. Begin cleansing your entire neck and behind your ears with gentle circular motions. Grime sticks to those areas like glue.

- Next, starting at the tips of your fingers, work your way up and around your arms, making sure that lather touches everything, including your elbows. Take more time and use a bit of extra pressure in your armpits, especially if you have hair there. After you finish one arm, resoap before you wash the other arm. Next, carefully scrub your breasts, making sure to wash underneath and between them.

- Move to your stomach, getting into your belly button (you might want to use a cotton swab), and start working on your back, making an effort to reach the center.

- Resoap and start lathering your tush. They don't call it a crack for nothing! As in any tiny area, tons of body gunk finds its way in there. To get clean, lift your legs one at a time and do some light scrubbing, making sure to resoap and rinse with clean water.

- The vulva is where washing gets tricky. All that hair and those folds make it a veritable fun house for funk, meaning you need to take extra care when cleaning it. You'll only need a little soap, and something gentle is best. Using harsh suds or using too much can irritate the delicate skin. With a small amount of soap on your fingertips, pull out your labia and gently hand wash each part individually. Be careful not to get soap in your vagina; it can irritate the inner membranes and cause pain.

- Rinse and resoap your washcloth; then start working your way down and around your legs. When you get to your feet, wash between your toes and spread the lather onto your soles. These areas can work up quite a funk while you're walking around all day.

- Rinse your entire body, washing off all leftover suds. Spread your bottom cheeks and the folds of your labia so you can easily rinse them, too.

- Towel off, getting into all the crevices you just cleaned. Apply enough deodorant to your underarms to get you through the day. If foot odor is a problem, pick up some foot powder at your local drugstore and apply that before putting on your socks.

If this doesn't do the trick, it might be your hair that's making you smell! Keeping your scalp and body hair clean is just as important as washing your body, as your head, underarms, and groin can be flytraps for funk. If you're comfortable, trimming or removing some body fuzz might help evict bacteria and funk from their hairy homes, especially underneath your arms. Check out the "How To: Shave Properly" on page 166 and "Hair Removal Methods" on page 173 for some tips.

## WHAT IF THEY NOTICE?

If you find yourself becoming a magnet for body musk as the day moves along, try keeping a travel-size stick of deodorant, some baby wipes, and perhaps a body fragrance with you so you can periodically freshen up.

# I'm addicted to tanning.

## WHAT'S GOING ON?

Tanning is a fun, social, and relaxing activity, which is why so many of us get caught up in this unhealthy obsession, especially if all our friends are into it, too.

Problem is, too much tanning can be D-E-A-D-L-Y. Why? As the Earth's ozone layer continues to deplete, tanners are being exposed to more and more of the sun's UV rays, making catching rays outside increasingly dangerous in recent years. Using a tanning bed is no safer. Concentrated rays sizzle into your skin during booth sessions, causing cancer just as do rays straight from the sun.

Everyone kinda knows that tanning is bad, but the tanning trend has still taken off. About 75 percent of teens prefer tan skin, with 89 percent of teen girls and 78 percent of boys saying they "actively pursue" a tan.

Skin cancer is a big problem for young adults. Melanoma is the most deadly kind of skin cancer, and it is now the most common cause of cancer death among women in their twenties. In the past, people suffering with the condition were usually fifty and older. The main cause of melanoma? You guessed it: baking in the sun or at the salon.

Because of the increase in skin cancer, the American Academy of Dermatology suggests that EVERYONE, regardless of skin type, use sunscreen with an SPF of at least 15 for the ENTIRE year. If you have many moles, close relatives with many moles, very fair skin and hair, or a family history of skin

## TAN-OREXIA
### WARNING SIGNS

*Do you . . .*

- go to tanning salons *and* lie out in the sun?
- use tanning as a stress reliever or as an escape?
- never feel tan enough?
- constantly worry about your tan fading?
- avoid sunscreen because it will lessen your tan?
- tan through body pain or headaches?
- ignore others when they say you're way too dark?
- lie at the tanning salon about your tanning history?

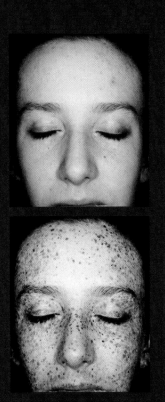

This teen girl is a chronic tanner. The top picture shows the outer skin layer we see when we look at her face: It appears to be clear and healthy. The bottom picture is a photograph taken under ultraviolet (UV) light. It shows the skin layer directly beneath what is normally visible. Check out the damage! While her epidermis looks medium well-done, the inside layers look overcooked. If she doesn't start taking some serious precautions in the sun, her outside will soon catch up with her inside.

cancer, use the highest SPF you can find (anywhere from SPF 20 up to SPF 45), cover up, and try to stay out of the sun. You're at higher risk for skin cancer.

Regardless of the death sentence, some people are really, really obsessed with their tans, to the point of being "tan-orexic." What's a tan-orexic? In the same way people with anorexia are obsessed with being thin and afraid of being fat, people suffering from tan-orexia are obsessed with being tan and fearful of being pale. The darker the tan, the more beautiful a person with tan-orexia feels.

## HOW DO I DEAL?

First, lay off the booth and turn to the spray for your tanning fix. See page 46 for tips on how to achieve the perfect fake bake. If you're very pale or if your skin tends not to take fake tanners well, try using bronzing makeup and tinting moisturizing lotions, both of which give you a great glow!

There's no excuse for tanning in a booth (EVER!) when you can safely buy your golden bake, but there are many fun reasons to go to the beach or pool, so be prepared. When you're bound for the outdoors, slather yourself with sunscreen, wear sunglasses, and don a cute floppy hat. Stay out of the sun during peak intensity times (usually somewhere between 10 A.M. and 3 P.M.) and do your best not to burn. Sunburns more than DOUBLE your risk for getting melanoma, especially if you burn your body when you're young. Check your entire body at least once a month.

*See your doctor immediately if*
- you answer yes to any of the ABCD questions (see facing page).
- you have any of the following: one mole or freckle that looks a lot different from the others, a scaly red spot, bleeding, or a sore on your body that refuses to heal.

Think you're off the skin cancer hook because you have darker skin? Not so fast! While it's much easier for fair people to get skin cancers, dark-skinned people get them, too. People of all ethnicities should check for potentially cancerous spots on the bottoms of feet, the skin between toes, underneath toenails, genitals, palms of their hands, and the insides of mouths and noses (if you can see in there!) once a month. Cancerous cells can pop up anywhere!

Skin cancer, when caught early, is treatable and beatable, so put your pride aside and *see your doctor* about that bothersome bump or tanning habit.

*fast fact*

*In the 1800s, being pale was considered a sign of nobility and class. Common people worked outdoors to earn a living and grow their food, while wealthier members of society remained pale because they could afford servants and did not have to work outside. With modernity causing a switch in common careers, tanning became popular in the 1920s when Coco Chanel started sporting the accidental "luxury tan" she got lounging in the sun all day instead of working inside.*

F.Y.I.

# DETECTING SKIN CANCER

**Is that mole or freckle cancerous? Know the ABCDs for detecting skin cancer:**

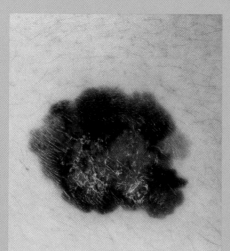

## A = ASYMMETRY
Are your body marks not the same shape and/or size all around?

## B = BORDER IRREGULARITIES
Do the edges look as if a kindergartner colored outside the lines?

## C = CHANGING COLORS
Is the spot brown one day, black another, or two-toned always?

## D = DIAMETER
Is it larger than a pencil eraser?

Tanning booths and extended sun sessions are off-limits, but you don't have to stay winter white. Here are three options for getting a great glow.

## DO IT YOURSELF SELF-TANNER

**COST:** cheap

**LASTS:** two to seven days

**PROCEDURE:** Taking tanning into your own hands? Here are some simple steps so that your skin looks superb and not streaky. When using a new product, always carefully read the directions to make sure you apply it correctly. If possible, self-tan with a friend. Having someone to reach those difficult spots (especially your back) will help prevent streaks.

① Exfoliate beforehand. That way, when you apply the self-tanner, patches of your tanned skin won't shed at different rates, leaving splotches.

② Moisturize before you begin, to help the tanning solution spread evenly and smoothly.

③ Working from your feet up, apply a thin coat quickly with an even hand. Rubbing the tanner in is not nearly as important as getting an even layer. Don't apply too much. It's easy to add more lotion if you want a deeper glow, but it's hard to reverse the process. Using a cloth or rubber glove is a good idea. There's nothing worse than a telltale glowing palm.

④ Use a makeup sponge or cotton ball to apply self-tanner to your face with light strokes. This procedure will help prevent irritation and streaking. Also, use a cotton swab to clean the tanner from your cuticles and nails after applying self-tanner to your hands. Destroy the evidence!

⑤ Wash your hands well and wait. The tanning solution will need time to sink in. Don't try to put on clothes, exercise, bathe, or do much of anything for at least a half hour after application. If you're in a hurry, use a hair dryer to speed up the process. Still, make certain your tan is set before getting dressed, or you'll make a mess!

If you feel as if you might have over fake-baked, exfoliating will help get your skin back to normal faster. If you want to go a little darker, try applying another even layer. Not satisfied with the results? There are many kinds of self-tanner out there, and different skin types can have different reactions to the fake bake, so experiment with different products until you find the one that's right for you.

**PROS:** It's inexpensive, and because you're in control, self-tanner can be applied or reapplied anytime, anywhere.

**CONS:** It's messy, error-prone, and not nearly as relaxing as when the professionals do it.

### PROFESSIONAL AIRBRUSH/SPRAY SELF-TANNING

**COST:** moderate

**LASTS:** five to fourteen days

**PROCEDURE:** Either a woman with a spray gun or an automated machine mists you all over with a solution that combines with the amino acids in your skin to make you tan.

**PROS:** It's easy to do, gives a natural color, and is an interesting experience.

**CONS:** The machine can cause streaks if it doesn't spray evenly. If there's a real person spraying you, not a machine, you may feel awkward saying, "Scuze me, I think you missed my left butt cheek. Can you go back over it again?"

### PROFESSIONAL SELF-TANNING

**COST:** expensive

**LASTS:** two to seven days

**PROCEDURE:** Expect to lie naked on a table with your private areas covered while the technician exfoliates your skin with a body scrub, rinses you off, and then rubs self-tanning cream evenly all over your body.

**PROS:** The professionals can easily get to all those hard-to-reach areas, keeping you streak-free. The relaxing body scrub is a plus, too.

**CONS:** The results don't last any longer than the at-home fake bake, and a professional job is expensive.

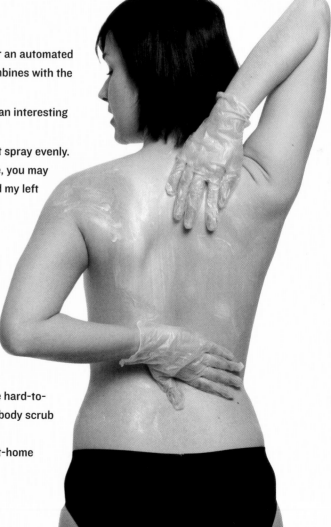

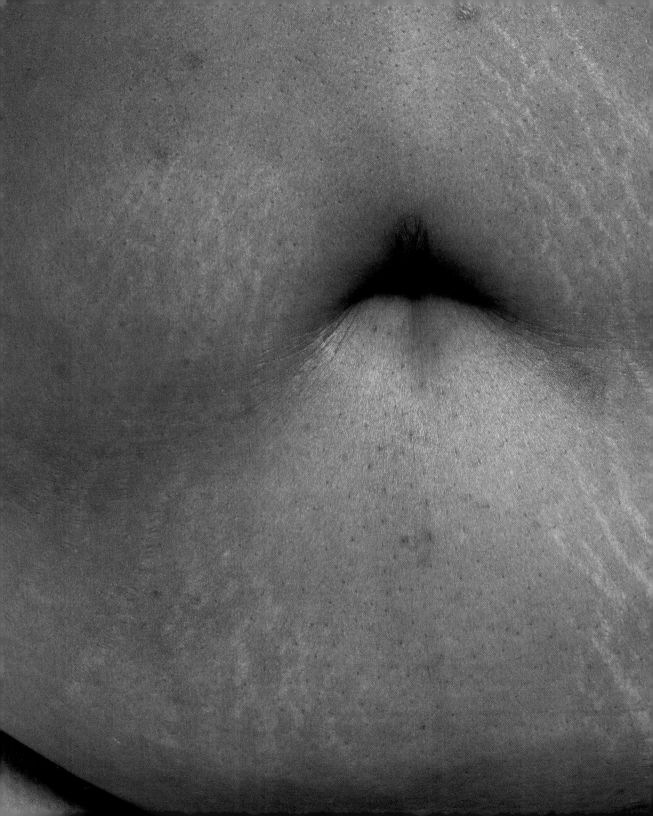

# My skin is full of stretch marks.

## WHAT'S GOING ON?

When your body goes through growth spurts or when you gain weight, the expansion can happen extremely fast. Sometimes it's so quick that your skin growth can't keep up, and your skin has to stretch very thin just to cover everything. This overstretching causes connective fibers in your skin to break and messes with your body's production of skin-supportive collagen, creating the road-map scars we call stretch marks. Although you can get stretch marks anywhere, they show up most frequently on hips, butt, thighs, arms, stomach, and breasts—all the places we're most obsessed with, right? Some people, such as those with drier skin or with a history of stretch marks in the family, are more prone to them than others.

## HOW DO I DEAL?

Stretch marks may look horrible to us when they first tarnish our treasured skin, but over time they gradually fade from reddish purple lines to a lighter, less noticeable color, sometimes disappearing altogether.

While you're waiting for them to fade, drink plenty of water, since stretch marks are minimized on hydrated skin. Although cocoa butter hasn't been proven to prevent or cure stretch marks, lotion lessens the look of skin lines, and cocoa butter is a cheap and fragrant way to stay soft and moisturized.

While there are medical procedures that claim to banish body bands, they don't work for everyone (sometimes the treatment may make the marks worse!) and can be very expensive.

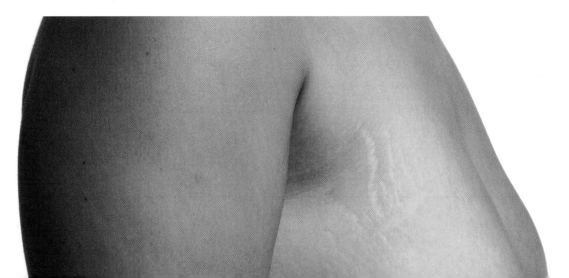

Still feeling zealous about concealing your zigzags? Certain brands of body makeup will stay put on your body parts, even in the pool! Also, with the right sunless tanning lotion, you can temporarily paint your stretch marks away. (Turn to page 46 to find out how to properly fake-bake).

## WHAT IF THEY NOTICE?

Nearly everyone has stretch marks, so don't worry too much. They're normal and have no negative impact on your health. If yours are from puberty, think of them as badges of honor or a rite of passage! Believe me, I wish there were more ways to get rid of or minimize them, but unfortunately, they're here to stay. With time, most of the marks will fade to become less of an issue.

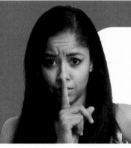

## i confess:
## i've bought scams from quacks

QUACK! QUACK! QUACK! NO, I didn't just randomly turn into a duck. I admit—I've wasted SO much money in the past on scams that promised to get rid of my cellulite, help me lose weight, immediately create a six-pack, grow my hair six to twelve inches in a month, and other absurd promises that I should have known were false. I always stared at the miraculous before and after photos, hoping that if it worked for those ladies, it would work for me! Even though the products never worked, I never blamed them—I blamed me. It wasn't until very recently that I found out that a lot of the products don't even work for the models that represent them.

For example, would you believe that a lot of cellulite cream ads take their before and after photos on the same day under completely different lighting? What's worse, a lot of the diet pill companies hire super-skinny models to take a photo for the after, gorge on food for a month, and come back to take the before!

So keep your cash in your checking account and your mind on self-improvement the good old-fashioned way—with diet, exercise, and self-confidence. Don't waste money like me—if it sounds too good to be true, then it probably is!

# Some parts of my body have darker skin than others.

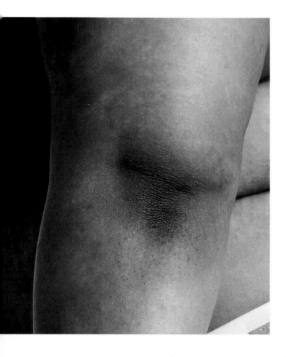

## WHAT'S GOING ON?

Are pigment problems making you pause before putting on a short skirt or sleeveless top? It's expected that a popped pimple might leave a skin mark, but what makes knees, elbows, and other body parts darker than the rest?

Most women, especially women of color, deal with natural variations in shade all over their bodies. The skin's coloration is determined by the pigment melanin, which is produced by cells called melanocytes (**muh-LAN-uh-sites**). We all have about the same number of melanocytes, but it's their activity, not how many exist, that matters most when determining skin pigmentation. The more active your melanocytes, the darker your skin becomes. Different situations excite your melanocytes into hyperactivity—sun exposure being one of them.

*Sometimes, melanocytes concentrate their action in a single area because of:*

- **Friction.** Constant pressure from toe-squeezing stiletto heels, inner thigh chafing, or too-tight bra straps creates melanocyte explosions.
- **Irritation.** Popping pimples, reckless shaving, cuts, bruises, and rashes all send signals for melanocytes to get busy.
- **Skin folds.** Places that naturally wrinkle and crease, such as your joints, invite melanocyte activity.

## HOW DO I DEAL?

It's common for some body parts to be darker than others, and although much of what determines the body's coloration is genetic, there are a few things you can do to avoid being TOO two-toned.

If you think your color variation might be caused by friction, try wearing bras or shoes that aren't as tight. Always lotion up, taking care to lubricate the darker spots heavily. Moisturized skin always looks healthier!

Are you determined to rid yourself of the dark spots you already have? Citric acid lightens skin because it helps to remove old layers of dead cells. Try scrubbing the areas regularly with 1 tablespoon sugar and 1 tablespoon lemon juice. ☀ **CAUTION:** DO NOT use this exfoliant on your face or genitals. It's too harsh for most of us and will seriously irritate your sensitive skin, potentially darkening the skin even more.

Fading creams, although they might lighten the skin, may also leave your skin permanently ashy and dull. Avoid them UNLESS under a doctor's supervision. Only a doctor can give you prescription-strength creams that are safe and effective.

*fast fact*

*Over 2 million Americans have a skin condition called vitiligo (vit'l-EYE-goh), where the melanocytes in some body parts die or become completely inactive. When this happens, areas of skin turn completely white, since pigment is no longer being produced. See your doctor if you start noticing depigmentation. There are treatments available to help you regain your color.*

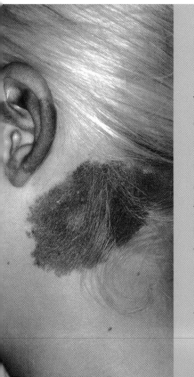

# BIRTHMARKS

Why are some people marked for life? No one can explain the precise cause of these spots of hyperpigmentation (darker marks on lighter skin) or hypopigmentation (lighter marks on darker skin), but genetics plays a part in the mix. Having a potato-shaped area on your arm or a map of Florida on your stomach serves as a great conversation piece, but it's not as easy to brush off a facial birthmark. In the past, birthmarks on the face were permanently disfiguring and impossible to conceal. Today, advanced laser technologies can remove many of them. Can't go under the laser just yet? Many makeup brands can perfectly blend the spot with the rest of your skin, no matter how different the two colorings may be! Visit www.nancyredd.com for some before and after birthmark shots.

F.Y.I.

# My skin is rough and dry.

## WHAT'S GOING ON?

Life is full of rough patches, but your skin shouldn't be among them!

The epidermis is the top layer of your skin, and its cells are glued together by an oily layer made of fat and cholesterol. This "glue" helps you retain your body moisture and blocks out most substances, nearly waterproofing your body. Despite that protective layer, our skin still loses a lot of water daily, and even more water escapes if the skin lacks lipids, leading to xerosis **(zih-ROH-sis)**, the medical term for dry skin.

Signs of xerosis include rough spots, scales, cracks, and cuts all over or in specific spots of your body. Xerosis in itself isn't threatening to health, but when left untreated, these scales and cracks can worsen into infections, scars, and other skin disorders.

## HOW DO I DEAL?

Although a lack of skin moisture causes dry, rough skin, water intake alone isn't enough to get rid of xerosis. Although water is crucial to preventing dehydration, soaking in the tub (as good as it feels) won't solve the problem. The water that soaks into your skin's outer layers during a bath evaporates shortly after you dry off, leaving you high and dry.

*If you're as scaly as a lizard, try these techniques to boost your body's natural oils, which will, in turn, soften your skin:*

**Cleanse carefully.** Always use lukewarm water to gently wash, not polish, your body. Harsh scrubbing and hot water dry the skin, allowing moisture to escape. Use softening soaps and avoid products with harsh chemical ingredients, such as alcohol.

**Moisturize.** Frequently use a good emollient-rich cream. Emollients help to conserve moisture and replace lipids by filling in skin cracks with a water-in-oil mixture, helping to seal the skin. Look for ingredients such as petroleum, paraffin, beeswax, cocoa butter, olive oil, and lanolin.

**Stay healthy.** Do you smoke or tan? You're drying your skin and shrinking your life span all at the same time. Smoking and tanning are skin nightmares, causing extreme dryness and premature wrinkling. They don't call it baking in the sun for nothing!

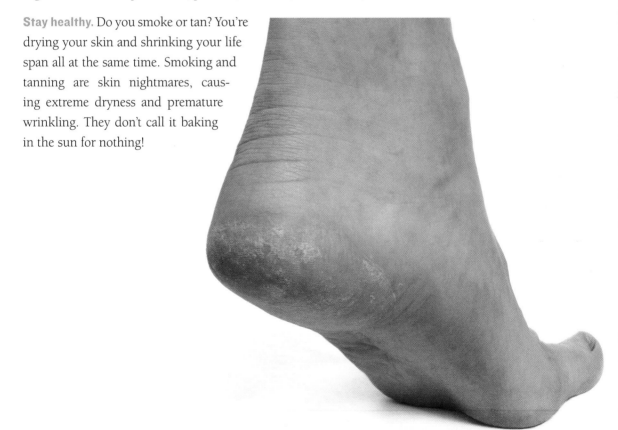

# My thighs look like cottage cheese.

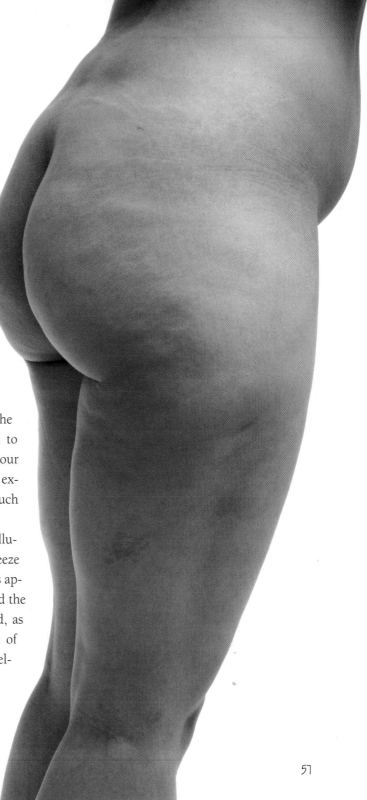

## WHAT'S GOING ON?

Dimples on your cheeks and chin are adorable, but when they show up on your butt and thighs, that's another story!

Cellulite rears its bumpy head when deposits of fat push against your skin's connective tissue, creating lumps on your skin's surface. No matter how sick you may feel about cellulite, orange-peel thighs aren't a disease, and since experts don't consider it a medical concern, there is no official doctor-speak for it.

Still, science has proven that the amount of cellulite you have is linked to genetics, age, diet, and exercise. So, if your mom has a bumpy butt or if you're not exercising and eating right, cellulite is much more likely to appear.

How do you know if you have cellulite? You can see it! If you're not sure, squeeze your stomach, thighs, or butt. Do ripples appear? If so, congratulations. You've joined the ranks of most women around the world, as *Newsweek* reports that over 85 percent of women over the age of eighteen have cellulite somewhere on their bodies.

## HOW DO I DEAL?

While creams, lasers, pills, and other products that claim to cut cellulite are wastes of money, there are ways you can reduce and camouflage cellulite. For starters, drinking enough water during the day helps to keep skin smooth. Dehydrated skin makes cellulite more apparent. Also, moisturized skin looks more toned and healthy than dry skin, so lotion up!

Exercise is a great skin solution, too. It won't get rid of cellulite, but lifting weights and doing cardiovascular work not only make you stronger and healthier, but also tighten and tone areas that are cellulite (and stretch mark) prone.

Although using a body brush or shower scrub won't get rid of cellulite, it will help your skin shine and glisten. Similarly, tanning can sometimes minimize the appearance of cellulite, but don't use dimpled skin as an excuse to bake in the tanning bed or in the sun without sunscreen. Opt for sunless tanning lotions or sprays to get the same effect.

## WHAT IF THEY NOTICE?

As big a deal as it may seem to you, your cellulite really isn't as noticeable to others, who are probably too busy stressing about their own butt lumps to pay attention to yours! If you're nervous about your cellulite being on display in a swimsuit, get a cute sarong coverup or wear a suit with boy-cut shorts. Remember, many swimsuit models have cellulite, too. It just gets airbrushed out before you get a chance to see it. (Turn to page 240 for more information.)

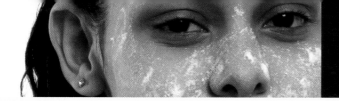

Gorgeous skin doesn't have to cost a fortune. You can beautify your skin with common household ingredients!

☀ CAUTION: Food and chemical allergies also apply to what you spread on the outside of your body. For example, if your throat closes when you eat avocados, **DO NOT** use the avocado facial mask. If you're allergic to aspirin, don't try the asprin mask on page 32.

Even if you don't have any allergies that you know about, it's a good idea to do a "patch test." Before using, dab some of the mask or scrub on your neck or inner wrist and wait five minutes to check for allergic reactions, such as redness, tingling, or a rash.

### HONEY-AVOCADO FACIAL MASK

*1/2 avocado*
*3 tablespoons honey*
*3 tablespoons plain yogurt*

Peel and chop the avocado into fine pieces. Mix thoroughly in a bowl with the honey and yogurt. Immediately spread over your face and neck, leaving on for five to ten minutes. Rinse. Avocado oil moisturizes while the yogurt hydrates and exfoliates. Honey is a mild antiseptic and helps to soothe and refresh your skin.

### CITRIC ACID FACIAL SCRUB

*1 orange*
*3 tablespoons regular oatmeal*

Slice the orange in half, squeezing its juices and pulp into a cup. Remove the seeds and add oatmeal until the mixture is spreadable. Apply to a clean face, and scrub gently. Rinse. Citric acid helps to loosen dead skin cells, while the oatmeal helps to slough them off, leaving you with glowing skin.

### COFFEE GROUNDS BODY SCRUB

*1 coffeepot*
*4 tablespoons ground coffee*
*2 tablespoons sugar*

Brew a pot of coffee as directed on your machine. Let the machine cool down for about ten minutes. Remove the grounds and mix them in a cup with the sugar. In the shower, use them as an invigorating body scrub. The caffeine in coffee grounds helps smooth and tighten skin for a short time.

For more masks, scrubs, and other do-it-yourself body recipes, check out www.nancyredd.com.

DRAMA #10

My piercing isn't healing well.

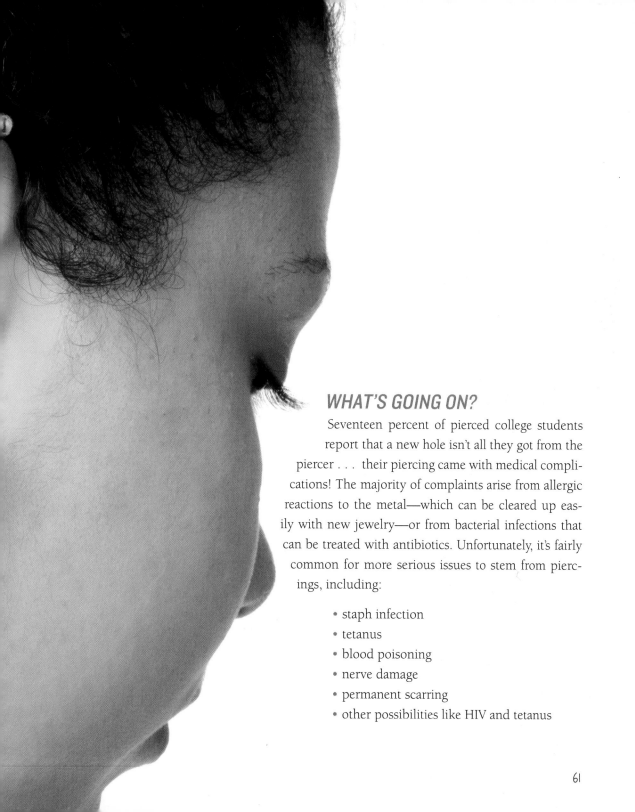

## WHAT'S GOING ON?

Seventeen percent of pierced college students report that a new hole isn't all they got from the piercer . . . their piercing came with medical complications! The majority of complaints arise from allergic reactions to the metal—which can be cleared up easily with new jewelry—or from bacterial infections that can be treated with antibiotics. Unfortunately, it's fairly common for more serious issues to stem from piercings, including:

- staph infection
- tetanus
- blood poisoning
- nerve damage
- permanent scarring
- other possibilities like HIV and tetanus

Common reasons for infection include perspiration, allergic reactions to metal, constant irritation from your clothes rubbing against the piercing, nonsterile piercing practices, and surface bacteria finding their way into the fresh wound. Signs of an infected piercing include:

- soreness
- redness
- swelling
- pain
- funny smells (yuk)
- dripping pus (double yuk, but common in infections)

But infections aren't the only complications that come with piercings. Other common piercing complications include:

- allergic reactions
- keloid formation
- jewelry migration or rejection
- tearing
- sores
- permanent numbness

Certain piercings carry even more severe consequences. A genital piercing may compromise condom use. The area with the most potential piercing complications? Your mouth. Complications

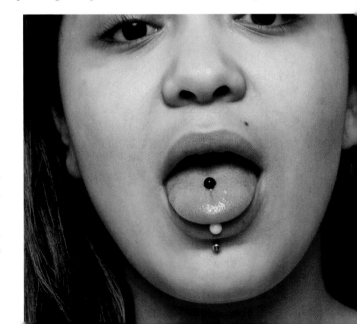

include all of the above, *plus* accidentally swallowing your jewelry, altered eating habits, injured salivary glands, loss of taste, speech impediments, tooth chipping and fractures, and uncontrolable drooling.

☀ **CAUTION:** Tongue rings (see right) have been linked to everything from chipped teeth to heart attacks, but recently, improperly placed rings have been found to cause a rare nerve disorder. It's called "suicide disease" because it's unbearably painful. In one case, a teenage girl suffered jolts of pain shooting through her body twenty to thirty times a day for months. Nothing helped until she removed her tongue piercing. The pain vanished two days later. Apparently, the tiny mouth barbell had been placed incorrectly and irritated a mouth nerve that connected, in turn, to a very important head nerve, causing the unbelievable pain.

## HOW DO I DEAL?

It's not just college students who are affected. As many as 35 percent of people with piercings suffer at least one complication during the healing process, so this is a common problem that shouldn't cause you shame. If a bit of smelly crust just popped up, the problem might be your personal hygiene habits. For up to a year after it is done, the piercing is an open wound, meaning your cleanliness needs to be ramped way up to ensure a healthy healing period and a pretty piercing. While some initial scabbing and bruising are normal after a piercing, if you're noticing other symptoms or if the spot doesn't seem to be healing, *see your doctor.*

Giving your piercing enough time to heal is very important in preventing infection. Want to bare that beautiful belly ring at the beach over the summer? You'll need to plan your navel piercing for September or October, for it can take up to nine months to mend properly. Here's a list of healing times.

| PIERCING | HEALING TIME |
|---|---|
| Navel | Up to nine months |
| Labia | Two to four months |
| Nipple | Two to four months |
| Nostril | Eight to ten weeks |
| Ear (lobe and upper) | Six to eight weeks |
| Mouth (lip or tongue) | Three to eight weeks |

### MOST POPULAR PIERCINGS

According to a recent study of college students, 51 percent of young women have more than just their earlobes pierced. Here are the most fashionable extra holes in order of popularity:

① navel
② ear (above the lobe)
③ tongue
④ nipple

Although it's a popular option, a mouth piercing is best avoided (see the facing page for why). If you do bite the bullet, unless you want a tongue the size of Texas, follow ALL the directions the piercer gives you and clean the piercing after EVERY meal.

The most important thing you can do for a healthy healing time is to stay dry and keep clean. The piercing should stay dry because moisture breeds infection-causing bacteria. That being said, to prevent scarring and pain, you should clean the piercing and turn the jewelry only when it's wet—preferably every time you're in the shower or just after you've bathed. Use a cotton swab to clean out all of the crevices.

While that belly ring might seem fun and carefree, piercings carry a lifetime of responsibility. If you suspect that yours isn't done properly or if you're having pain, pus, or other problems with your piercing, *see your doctor immediately*. If you let the infection go unchecked, you could develop serious health problems. Often, pierced people don't want to seek treatment for their infection because they fear that the doctor will tell them to take the piercing out. Problem is, an infection probably won't go away by itself, and chances are it will only worsen. Ask yourself: Would you rather lose your piercing or your tongue?

F.Y.I.

# KELOIDS

Remember that a piercing or tattoo is really just a wound. Your body knows this and makes a sincere effort to heal itself, not knowing you paid money to have the injury done deliberately. In some people, especially women of color, the body is determined to heal the wound once and for all, going into overdrive and creating keloids, mounds of itchy, thick, puckered, and disfiguring scar tissue that surround the wound. Keloids can also pop up from other cuts and lesions, but until a keloid grows on you, there's no way to know if you're keloid-prone. If someone in your family suffers from keloids, you may want to rethink your piercing. If you are still interested, *talk to your doctor* first, who may be able to offer medicine to help you avoid the scars.

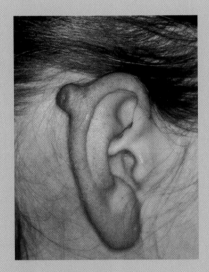

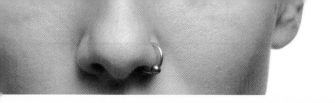

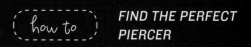
Feel the need for a new hole in your head? Here's how to choose when, where, and how you are pierced to make sure the result draws envious stares and not repulsed glares.

**Have enough cash** to get your piercing done in a safe, clean place. The time to economize is NOT when you're deciding on a piercer. Factoring in the proper body jewelry, antiseptic, and the piercer's time and expertise, a new piercing will create a new dent in your body AND in your wallet.

**Ask to see a book of the piercer's work** and confirm that the photos are of piercings actually done by the person who will be working on you. Sadly, higher prices don't guarantee quality.

**Make sure your piercer has a license to practice** and is not just some wannabe with a needle and an ice cube. You could get a SERIOUS infection.

**Get recommendations** from friends and people whose piercings look good and have healed properly. If possible, watch the piercer work on someone else, noting his or her cleanliness. If your piercer doesn't practice perfect sterilization (a new needle, clean gloved hands), there is a chance you could get an infection such as tetanus or hepatitis B or C from a dirty needle.

**Be patient.** If you can't find someone you can afford and feel comfortable with, wait until you can. Who knows, by the time you're ready, the trend may have changed, or YOU may have changed your mind about this fashion statement.

And depending on where you live, you might *have* to settle for a stick-on or magnetic fake piercing for now. Most piercing establishments in the United States require that a parent or guardian be present or sign for you to get pierced, and many states have laws against body piercing for people under eighteen, regardless of what their parents think. The government isn't trying to ruin your fun; the laws are there to protect you. If you pierce the skin of an area that's still growing, such as your torso (belly button) or nose (yes, your nose continues to grow), there's a chance that your piercing might stretch as well, causing a disgusting deformity.

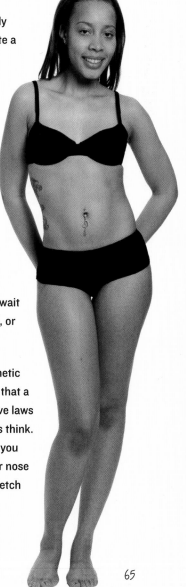

# SAFE TATTOOING

Are you deciding whether to try a tattoo? Before you get started, make sure you're ready. Once inked in, tattoos are expensive and difficult—sometimes impossible—to remove. Possible complications of tattooing include hepatitis, bacterial and viral infections, general skin irritation, allergy to the ink used, and disfigurement. These issues are common even in professional environments where safety precautions are standard. The risks jump much higher if you attempt to tattoo yourself or have a friend do it. There's NO WAY you can get a do-it-yourself tattoo safely, no matter how many times your friends say they have done it.

## *BEFORE* YOU GET A TATTOO:

- Check that your tattoo artist is licensed and ask to see proof.

- Check the artist's portfolio. If you're in the market for a smiling cartoon butterfly, a tattoo artist who specializes in realistic vampires might not be your best bet, no matter what assurances he or she gives you.

- Ask if the tattoo artist sterilizes their equipment with an autoclave. An autoclave is the only machine capable of heating tattooing equipment high enough to sterilize them. See if you can watch the sanitizing process to make certain your tools are clean.

- Look around. Does the shop look clean, well-lit, and safe? If not, choose somewhere else to get your artwork done.

- Be prepared for pain. Some people handle it better than others, but find out beforehand how long the procedure will take so you can pace yourself (or chicken out)!

## *AFTER* YOU GET A TATTOO:

- NO TOUCHING, no matter how awesome it looks, for at least twenty-four hours. The bandage needs to stay on to help the fresh wound heal.

- After the first twenty-four hours, apply antibiotic ointment gently and often. Your tattoo artist should have sent you home with some. If not, get some at the drugstore.

- If scabs appear, don't pick them. You might ruin your design and cause scarring.

- Keep your tattoo dry and out of direct sunlight until it fully heals. Fading isn't the only reason to do so. Any open wound is a serious candidate for skin damage.

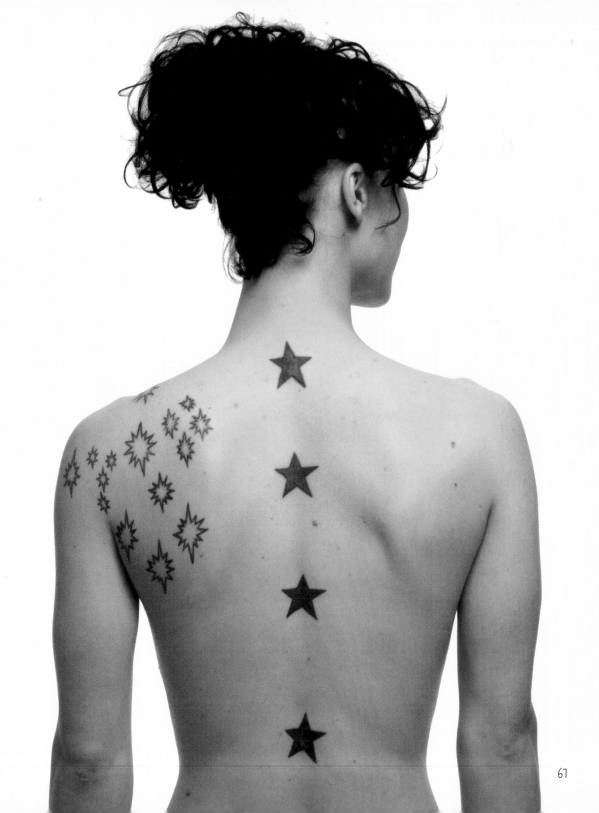

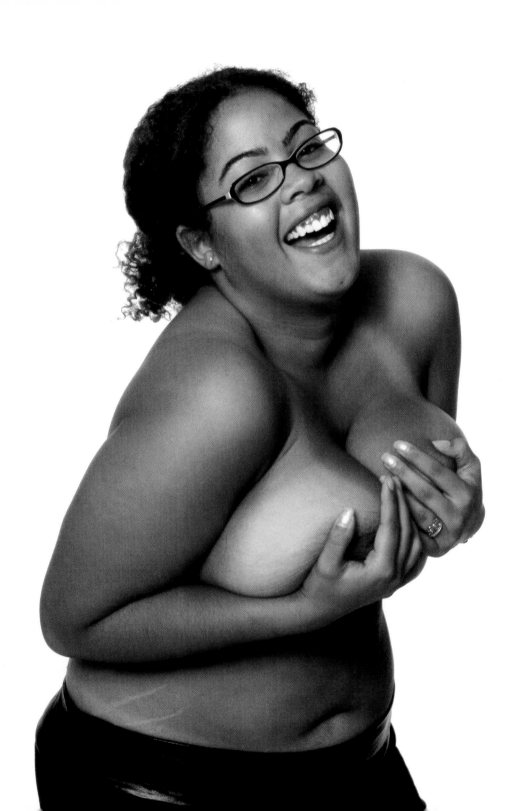

# BOOBS

I don't know about you, but in high school I always felt as if I missed the boat in the boob department. Since all the drawings and pictures I saw of breasts made them look like round, firm balls decorated with pencil erasers, my saggy cones with silver-dollar nipples didn't seem fair. My friend Zee had the largest breasts I'd ever seen—bigger than her head—and she hated hers, too, strapping them down 24/7 with two sports bras. Then there was Allie, whose chest was so flat she didn't even have to wear a bra during track practice! All three of us were concerned and confused by what was (or wasn't) going on right under our noses. What were these chest ornaments for, and why did we have to deal with them now? Even today I don't have an answer, and neither does anyone else: Humans are the only species to develop breasts long before they're needed to nurse babies, and scientists around the world are still trying to figure out why.

Most bets (both scientifically and between us girls) are that breasts enhance sexual arousal (for both males and females) and that, since humans went from walking on all fours to standing upright, breasts take the place of the buttocks and encourage communication (less likely, but still possible). Instead of waiting for the final press release, my friends and I have simply decided to invest in some good bras and work with what we have. Zee has started wearing a regular bra (and only one of them at a time), and Allie, much to her surprise, sprouted a solid B-cup in her junior year of college. So remember: Whatever boob drama you're going through, you're not alone. Just hang tight and read this chapter for tips on how to deal!

*Externally, your breasts are made up of nipples, areolas (the darkened skin around the nipples), and skin. Inside are milk glands, milk ducts, connective tissue, and fat.*

*Breasts begin developing while you're in your mother's womb. They just lie flat until puberty. Breast growth can continue well into your twenties.*

*Your mom might sport a C cup, but this doesn't mean that you'll be able to swap bras with her. Breast size can be inherited from both sides of your family.*

*Having a baby will probably temporarily increase your cup size (more room for milk storage) and darken your nipples.*

# I have no breasts at all.

## WHAT'S GOING ON?

There's a 99.9 percent chance that you DO have breasts! Even if you're as flat as a board, the area underneath your nipple contains all of the components of a healthy breast: milk glands, milk ducts, fat, and connective tissue. Externally, however, you may not have been blessed with the overflowing bosom you expected. Puberty is supposed to bring on an increase of fat in the breast area and an explosion of breast tissue. Although the growth sometimes happens as early as nine or ten years old, occasionally it doesn't happen until much later or not at all. For some women, the nipple may go through the first process of darkening and enlarging without the breast moving on to step two (growing!), even though all the other signs of maturity—such as pubic hair and menstruation—are visible. Still, don't stock up on a lifetime supply of AA cups just yet. Many young women have experienced seemingly overnight bosom bursts when they least expected them!

## HOW DO I DEAL?

Breasts are usually the first thing to sprout, but sometimes they're last on your body's to-do list. If you're worried about having "just" an A or a B cup, don't be. Though your melons may not be as ripe as your friends' are, they're still marvelous! Happen to be one of the thousands of young women who are a double-A or triple-A cup? Try not to stress, because regardless of your breasts' size, as long as all of your other signs of maturity are on track, you're completely normal and healthy. And, if you ever decide to have a baby, you'll still be able to breast-feed, because that has nothing to do with cup size. As a bonus, all that milk production will cause your boobs to grow—if only for a while!

For some young women the hormones in birth control pills cause breasts to grow bigger. This isn't true for every girl, though, and more important, it's not reason enough to begin taking hormones. And don't be fooled into purchasing expensive creams and pills that promise breast growth. These scams don't work and are a waste of time and money—and are sometimes dangerous!

No matter what your friends tell you, sleep positions, breast massages, and specific foods and drinks have no influence on your breasts' growth. What can affect their size, however, are your diet and eating habits. If you're on the slender side, diet constantly, or eat poorly, your body might not be getting enough of the nutrients and calories you need to grow breasts.

Still despairing over your indented chest? You don't have to sit back and twiddle your thumbs in anticipation of the boob fairy: A padded bra or inserts can magically fill out your clothes and swimsuits. Or you might decide that "faking it" is a waste of time and effort and revel in being able to jog without having to wrap your arms around your chest for support! If you do decide to stuff, keep an eye on your padding to make sure it stays in the right place (double-sided tape attached to your bra and the stuffing works wonders), since the slightest shift can give you the appearance of a third boob or even a hunchback!

## WHAT IF THEY NOTICE?

In a society obsessed with breasts, of course you feel frustrated if you're batting zero in the game of chest. If shallow people make fun of your somewhat shallow chest, know that they are the ones with the problem. You may feel tempted to wear oversize clothing and keep your distance from other people in hopes your flat chest will go unnoticed. Although such tactics may help you avoid the issue, you might miss a lot of fun, making you feel even worse. Don't allow your breasts (or lack thereof) to affect your self-esteem. Plenty of actresses, athletes, and other amazing women have and love their A-cup chests! Your boobs are only two of the hundreds of things that make you beautiful and unique!

| THE REAL MEANING OF BRA CUP SIZES | |
|---|---|
| A | Almost boobs |
| B | Barely boobs |
| C | Can't complain |
| D | Dang! |
| DD | Double Dang! |
| E | Enormous |
| F | Fake |
| G | Get a reduction |
| H | Help me, I've fallen and can't get up |

# 99 NICKNAMES FOR BOOBS

| | | | |
|---|---|---|---|
| Ant Bites | Elephants | Lung Covers | Sweater Puppets |
| Appalachians | Flotation Devices | Melons | Ta-tas |
| Apples | Fly Swatters | Mole Hills | Teacups |
| Altars | Fog Lights | Mosquito Bites | Tetas |
| Assets | Gland Canyon | Mountain Peaks | Twin Peaks |
| Baby Feeders | Girls | Nipple Caddies | Twofers |
| Backbreakers | Goodies | Nubbins | Udds |
| Bazoombas | Grand Tetons | Pencil Erasers | Umbrellas |
| Bitties | Gumdrops | Pillows | Umlauts |
| Bookends | Guns | Pom-Poms | Voos |
| Buds | Hood Ornaments | Puppies | Victrolas |
| Bumpers | Hooters | Pyramids | Volcanoes |
| Buoys | Hot Air Balloons | Quakers | Windbags |
| Buffoons | Hubcaps | Quantum Heaps | Womanhood |
| Buttons | Hush Puppies | Rack | Wonder Twins |
| Chestnuts | Hypnotizers | Raisins | Wongas |
| Coconuts | Igloos | Rib Cushions | Wookies |
| Cupcakes | Itty Bitties | Rockets | Xenoliths |
| Cushions | Jahoobies | Rosebuds | Yabbas |
| Doorknobs | Jugs | Shock Absorbers | Yahoos |
| Double Trouble | Jumblies | Snow Cones | Yeast Dough |
| Dumplings | Knockers | Sopapillas | Zeppelins |
| Earmuffs | Kumquats | Speed Bumps | Zingers |
| Eggs, Sunny Side Up | Love Handles | Sugar Plums | Zoombas |
| El Primo Torpedoes | Low Riders | Sultanas | |

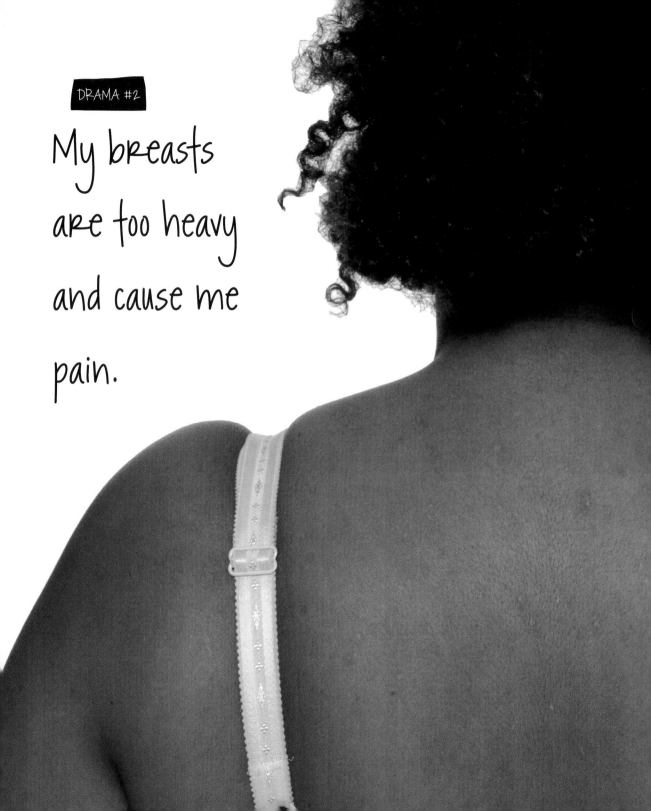

My breasts are too heavy and cause me pain.

## WHAT'S GOING ON?

Some women wish they had a bigger rack, while others want to put some back! Having big breasts can be a huge pain—literally. From back pain to shoulder grooving to skin rashes to posture problems, boobs that are extremely big in proportion to your frame and not properly supported can cause medical problems, not to mention self-consciousness. You may even experience headaches, breathing problems, skeletal damage, or other personal traumas due to your load!

## HOW DO I DEAL?

When your bra bulges with bigger boobs than everyone else's, people's reactions can be annoying. There's nothing worse than a face-to-chest conversation, and people—even your best friends—often feel that it's perfectly fine to comment on a very private part of your body.

It's simple to try to hide your big'uns by hunching your back, slouching your body, slumping your shoulders, or wearing oversize clothing—but just because it's easy doesn't mean it's right. These techniques might hide your large breasts a little bit, but they can hurt you in ways ranging from increased back pain to decreased self-esteem. And surprise: Having good posture and wearing clothes that fit will enhance your figure and appearance more than trying to mask your size. Looking better on the outside will help you feel better on the inside, both physically and mentally. Hold your head (and your chest) high and proud, and don't let other people's stares or your own stress bring you down.

## STRENGTHEN YOUR BACK

Lie facedown with your arms at your side. Keeping your legs tightly together and on the ground, slowly raise your chest off the floor as high as you comfortably can. Hold for two seconds and return to the beginning position. Do this for up to twenty times in a row and your back (and boobs) will thank you.

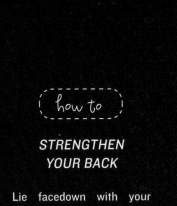

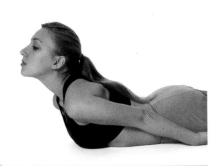

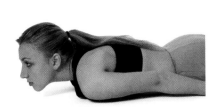

While no exercise will decrease the size of your breasts, weight loss may affect their size—but only if you have weight to lose in the first place. If you're already thin with large breasts, sorry, but they're probably here to stay. Strengthening your back with exercises (like the one to the left) won't shrink your boobs, but it will make you stronger, improve your posture, and diminish your pain.

Now that you're standing tall and strong, keep it that way with the proper bra! A great-fitting bra can minimize pain, rashes, shoulder grooving, and other boob-related ailments. These bras, appropriately called minimizers, play down the size of your breasts, drawing the attention up from your chest toward your fantastic face. Check out "Find a Bra That Fits" (page 92) and head to a good department or lingerie store where a knowledgeable salesperson can help you choose the bra that's right for you. Look for one with padded shoulder straps for extra comfort.

Warning: Bras for larger breasts, especially those that support and minimize, can be expensive. Many cost twice as much as a smaller bra, and some cost even more. If money's tight, *see your doctor,* who may vouch for the fact that you need a good bra so your health insurance will cover it. You might even qualify for a custom-designed medical bra!

Finally, if your breasts are completely out of control and cannot be tamed with a bra, good posture, and back exercises, a plastic surgeon can reduce them for you. Breast reduction usually isn't performed until adulthood, but exceptions are made for young women with serious medical issues, like the nineteen-year-old girl on the facing page, who went from a DDD to a C!

Would you rather look like this?

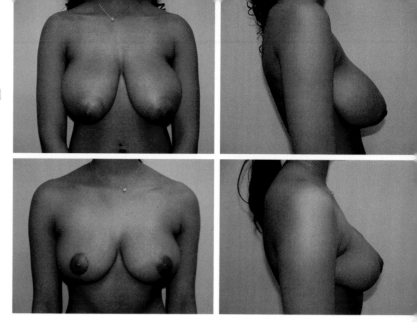

In this nineteen-year-old's case, the surgeon removed nearly a pound of fat from each of her breasts!

As you can see, breast reduction is serious surgery. It's not meant to make your breasts perfect-looking; rather, it is an option to improve the health of larger-breasted women. The procedure can leave you with scarring and less sensitivity. Still, it can help you feel better, and some health insurance plans cover the surgery. If you're in need of extreme relief, *see your doctor* for an evaluation.

## WHAT IF THEY NOTICE?

You control your breasts . . . don't let your breasts control you! Try not to feel self-conscious about your large breasts. If other people offend you, speak up! Tell them that their remarks make you feel uncomfortable and that their gibes are neither appropriate nor fair. Don't apologize for your boobs, make fun of them, or talk nasty about them. Regardless of their size, they're a huge part of you.

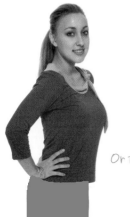

Or this?

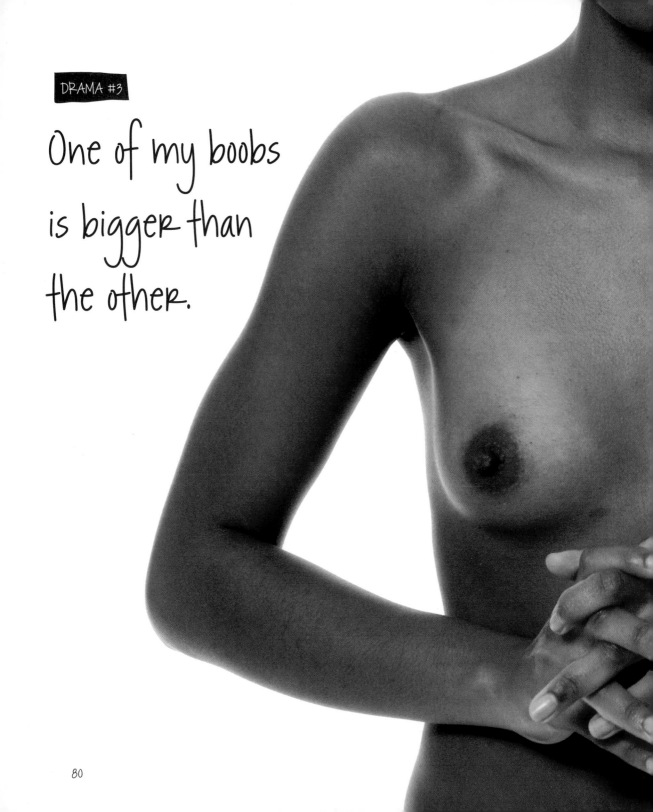

One of my boobs
is bigger than
the other.

80

## WHAT'S GOING ON?

Did you know that Ashley Olsen is an inch taller than her twin, Mary-Kate? That's because it's virtually impossible for two things to grow at exactly the same rate! One side of your hair grows faster than the other, and one of your arms is probably slightly longer. When you're checking your boobs in the mirror, you may get upset if your body appears lopsided. Don't be. Your left boob is probably larger than your right. Even if the difference is minimal, the left breast usually has more tissue in it. No one knows why, but every woman has breasts that are different from each other in some way, whether one nipple is larger, one breast is rounder, or one boob is bigger. In fact, size differences are so common that many bra straps are easily adjustable to fit different-size breasts!

## HOW DO I DEAL?

If one of your boobs is bigger than the other, be patient. In time the smaller breast may more or less "catch up" to the larger one, although some size difference will probably remain. If the difference is extreme, like in the picture on the facing page, *see your doctor.* Otherwise, spend time finding a bra that is comfortable and that fits your body (check out "Find a Bra That Fits," page 92). If you feel the need, you can always pad the side that is smaller, adjust your bra straps on each side for a better fit, or remove the padding from the side that is bigger if your bra has removable pads.

*fast fact*

**Nearly 500 million bras are sold in America each year, with sales totaling over $5 billion. That's a multitude of covered boobs!**

## WHAT IF THEY NOTICE?

Your breasts might never be exactly the same, but relax. Hardly anyone (if anyone!) will notice when you have your clothes on, so don't let your boob size affect your personality. If someone says something, remember this: Everyone has body issues. Ask those teasers about their body quirks! More than likely, they have issues they're frustrated about, too.

If romance is on your mind, don't forget: The person you're making out with is probably excited about the very idea of breasts. In the heat of things, no one is going to notice a bit of difference (as long as you don't bring it up).

F.Y.I

# A BRIEF (HA HA) **BRA** HISTORY ...

The corset originated about 2000 B.C., but brassieres ("bras" for short) have a shorter history. In 1910, Mary Phelps Jacob, a popular New York socialite, was planning to wear a sheer gown to an event and was dissatisfied with the undergarment options available to her. With the help of her maid, she sewed two handkerchiefs together, added some ribbon for straps, and wowed her friends. Mary patented her invention in 1914, and her bras became as hot back then as Victoria's Secret's are today. After some time, Mary wanted to go back to partying. She sold her bra patent to Warner Brothers Corset Company for only $1,500. Over the next thirty years, the company earned more then $15 million from her bra pattern!

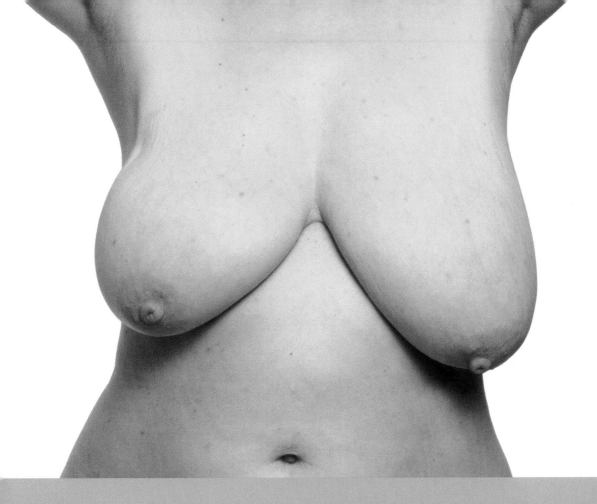

# ...AND THE HISTORY OF **NIPPLE PIERCING**

Do you think nipple piercing is something our generation came up with just to tick off the 'rents? Think again! Rumor has it that Cleopatra had an inverted nipple that she pierced to "coerce" it out, and Victorian doctors highly recommended piercing as a way to increase the size of nipples to make breast-feeding easier. Western women have been piercing their nipples for cosmetic reasons since the mid-fourteenth century, and in the past, they even wore special garments to show off the jewelry.

# My breasts are too far apart and I don't have any cleavage.

## WHAT'S GOING ON?

Nothing makes the "breasts are for arousal" argument more convincing than the human obsession with cleavage. Cleavage is the exposure of the vertical line that breasts create when they're smooshed together, either naturally or by the force of a powerful bra. The boob crack was popularized in the late fifteenth century when women started to wear corsets that flattened the stomach and lower part of the breast while pushing everything else up, up, up! This not only created lots of cleavage but also caused extreme discomfort and serious health consequences. Today, thank goodness, women get a rise out of their boobs mostly with push-up bras.

Surprisingly, your level of cleavage doesn't depend on your breast size or shape, but on how your boobs are positioned on your rib cage. The width of your rib cage and how it tilts determine how much of a line you can create. Because of varying rib cage inclinations, some women with large breasts find it difficult to create cleavage, while some small-breasted women have ribs that naturally tilt in toward their breastbone, which makes natural cleavage, even without a bra.

## HOW DO I DEAL?

Here's a test: How many fingers can you put vertically in the space between your breasts? The more fingers you can fit, the more difficulty you might face in your attempt to create a cleavage crack. Clearly, cleavage isn't a life or death situation, but if you want to enhance nature for a special occasion, check out the push-up bras in the lingerie store, as Sara did on page 88. You'll have to try on a few different ones before you find a bra that works without causing other problems (see page 92 for troubleshooting tips), but you'll certainly be able to find one that gives you a lift!

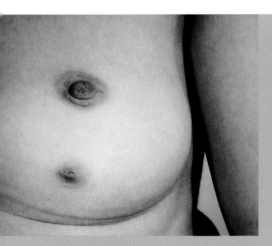

# THIRD NIPPLES

Do three make a crowd on your chest? Up to 5 percent of women have "accessory" nipples, medically known as polythelia and commonly referred to as a third nipple. Many people can mistake a strategically placed body mole for a third nipple, but when you see a real one (as in the picture here) you can tell the difference immediately. Third nipples usually appear along one of the two vertical milk duct lines in the breast, and they can take many forms, from a vague tuft of hair to a fully functioning, milk-producing nipple—perfect if you ever have triplets! Women are more prone to third nipples than men, and the incidence varies by ethnicity. As many as 5 percent of Japanese women have accessory nipples, compared to 3.5 percent of black women and fewer than I percent of Caucasians.

If you have an accessory nipple, don't freak out. As you can see from the statistics, it's fairly common. Still, schedule an appointment with your doctor if the extra nipple isn't already charted on your health history. Although the biggest drama with extra nipples might seem merely cosmetic, scientists have recently linked the gene for extra nipples to certain medical disorders. People with three or more nipples may be more prone to kidney disease, and scientists are looking into possible links between the gene for polythelia and breast cancer.

If you think your extra nipple might have to go, *talk to your doctor* about options. While the removal of accessory nipples is possible, the timing and conditions must be right to prevent scarring.

# My breasts aren't perky enough and/or don't bounce.

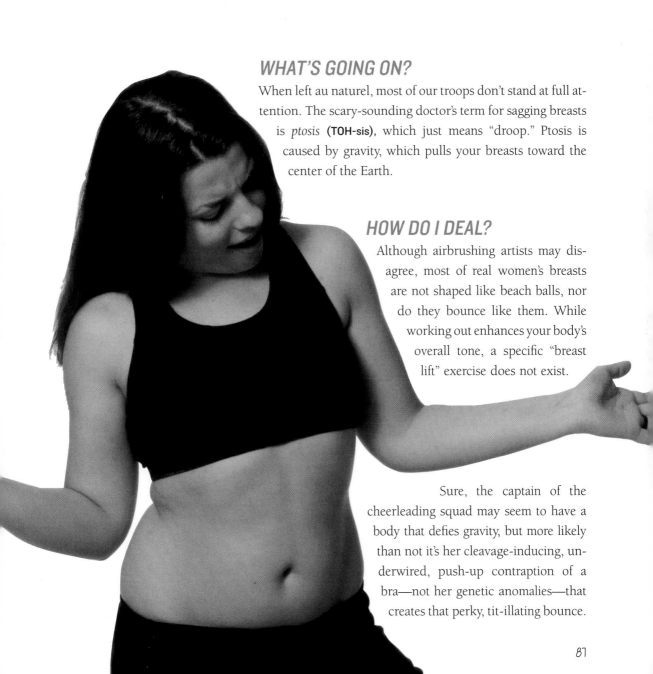

### WHAT'S GOING ON?

When left au naturel, most of our troops don't stand at full attention. The scary-sounding doctor's term for sagging breasts is *ptosis* **(TOH-sis)**, which just means "droop." Ptosis is caused by gravity, which pulls your breasts toward the center of the Earth.

### HOW DO I DEAL?

Although airbrushing artists may disagree, most of real women's breasts are not shaped like beach balls, nor do they bounce like them. While working out enhances your body's overall tone, a specific "breast lift" exercise does not exist.

Sure, the captain of the cheerleading squad may seem to have a body that defies gravity, but more likely than not it's her cleavage-inducing, underwired, push-up contraption of a bra—not her genetic anomalies—that creates that perky, tit-illating bounce.

In fact, the proof is in any bra catalog! Check out the photographs below to see what happens to Sara's girls in two different bras that are the same size. Certain bras designed to lift and squish can enhance your assets with no effort on your part. Turn to page 92 to learn how to choose the perfect bra for you.

Turn to page 92 to learn how to choose the perfect bra for you.

*fast fact*

*Nearly one-third of American women have size D cup or larger breasts. That's not a small fact to carry around. D cup breasts can weigh anywhere from fifteen to twenty-three pounds.*

## WHAT IF THEY NOTICE?

If you're worried about what you look like topless to romantic partners, know that when aroused, your nipples contract and the breasts become firmer, leading to a rounder look. If you're not aroused, then you shouldn't be baring your bod—but that's a whole other book!

F.Y.I.

# WHAT A DIFFERENCE A BRA MAKES!

Check out twenty-year-old Sara's boobs in two different types of bras, both size 38C. On the left, she's wearing a "regular" underwire bra, designed specifically for comfort and support. On the right, she's wearing a bra specifically designed to push breasts up and together, creating cleavage. What a difference! Depending on the type of bra, boob bounce can disappear and reappear faster than Houdini.

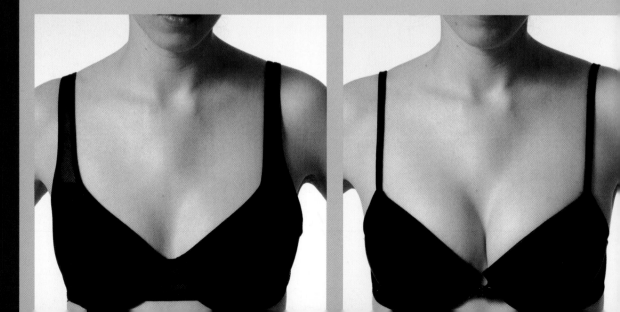

# CULTURAL CHEST PAINS

The way our breasts look and how they make us feel might stress us out at times, but that's nothing compared to how their appearance affects the education and freedom of hundreds of thousands of young women around the world. In villages in Cameroon, Africa, for example, citizens look to this age-old sign of puberty as a signal that a girl is maturing into a fertile young woman. To Cameroonians, breasts represent that a girl, no matter her age, is ready to be removed from school, leave her parents, take on a husband, and start a family of her own. Once removed from school, she will never be able to return. This renders her unskilled, illiterate, and capable only of working low-paying, tiring, and often demeaning jobs, all while raising a family. Since breasts can begin to appear at any time, many girls as young as seven or eight are married off to older men.

As Western customs trickle into Cameroon and as education becomes more widely available, many mothers, wanting to protect their girls from an impoverished fate, use an effective but grueling and destructive technique to delay their girls' breast growth—breast ironing. The act of breast ironing begins by heating a large stone, coconut shell, or other hard object in a fire. Then, the object is harshly rubbed and pounded against a young girl's chest, burning the area, destroying the connective tissue, and flattening the breast. This is repeated continually throughout puberty in an attempt to keep the girl in school. Up to 26 percent of girls suffer this painful ironing, at the hands of someone who loves them and just wants the best for them and their future. Sadly, some girls, desperate for a future, resort to self-ironing.

Efforts are being made to raise awareness in these villages about the dangers of breast ironing, and efforts are also being made toward stopping the appearance of breasts from being the determining factor for when girls should marry.

Even though breasts are "tops" in Western culture when it comes to sexual appeal, we are fortunate that for us, unlike our Cameroonian sisters, they don't affect our future in this way. For more information on breast ironing and how to help women in need, visit www.nancyredd.com.

My nipples are always hard.

## WHAT'S GOING ON?

Nipplage is the interesting phenomenon in which one's erect nipples are visible through clothing. It's rumored that a certain celeb employed assistants to ice her nipples to maintain her nipplage during the production of one of her music videos! Besides intentional icing, nipplage can be caused by a variety of factors such as cold weather, sexual interest, or friction against one's clothing. Sometimes nature simply likes to turn on your headlights at the most inopportune times and for no reason at all—which can lead to both physical and mental irritation.

## HOW DO I DEAL?

When you don't want two mosquito bites on your chest in your way, there are many simple ways to minimize nipplage. One easy way is to layer your clothing. More fabric gives you more coverage and control, so if your nipples have a tendency to pop out without notice, keep an extra top handy and pop it on over your clothes at the first sign of nipple-popping. Another simple solution is to check your bra. If it's made of thin material, try inserting more padding or buying a bra with cups made of thicker material. If you're going braless, carefully applied Band-Aids can help mask the mounds for half the price of the boobie covers (made for the same purpose) sold in stores. Make sure to cover your nipple with the nonadhesive part, and when it's time to remove, pull slooooooowly. Moisturize the area afterward to help it recover. DO NOT use duct tape, electrical tape, double-sided tape, or other strong adhesives. While your enthusiastic nipples might be causing you grief, there's no reason to punish them (or you) by accidentally ripping them off!

*fast fact*

*Nearly all women have nipple hair. It's just more noticeable on some than others. If you want to get rid of it, you can have it professionally waxed, or you can pluck it (carefully) with tweezers. You shouldn't spend too much time fretting, though, as a little chest hair is normal. For more information on stray strands, see page 170.*

## WHAT IF THEY NOTICE?

While nipplage may cause a few stares when it happens, there's nothing abnormal about erect nipples (it happens to men, too), so try not to worry. Some companies even sell fake rubber nipples that you can put on underneath your clothes, so some women can always have that "cold room" look. Indeed, many women actively pursue nipplage, believing that it makes them more irresistible.

# FIND A BRA THAT FITS

Your bra should behave like a good friend: supportive, pleasant to be with, and uplifting. And, like a best friend forever (BFF), a bra should never make you hurt or feel uncomfortable. Yet most of us go through life wearing the equivalent of our worst enemies on our chests!

The average woman owns about six bras, and most of them probably don't fit well. The key to a good-fitting bra is matching your chest size (band) and breast size (cup) to the right bra. Considering that cup sizes range from AAAA to EE and beyond, and that band sizes range from thirty to fifty inches around (and higher), properly fitting a bra is not easy, which is why millions of women are walking around in bad bras. Common bra disasters include:

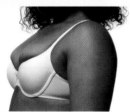

### THE PUCKERER
*If your bra cups have folds and wrinkles in them, your cup size is too big. Move down a size or two (such as from a B cup to an A cup) until the puckers are gone. If one of your cups puckers but the other fits fine, try adding a bit of padding or adjusting the straps on the puckering side.*

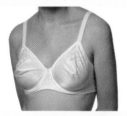

### THE PUSHER
*If your boobs are bulging out over the top of your bra, your cup size is too small or the cut of the bra is too low for your boobs. Go up a size or try a style with fuller coverage.*

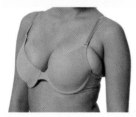

### THE PINCHER
*If your bra cuts into the side of your breast, your band size is probably too small, or you may have chosen a bra with sides that are too narrow for your frame. If the problem still happens with your hooks on the widest settings, go up a band size, and look for bras that have wider sides or bands for added comfort.*

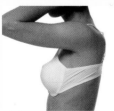

### THE RIDER
*If your bra rides up your back instead of resting at the same level all around your chest, your band size is probably too big. Either hook your bra on a tighter setting and loosen the straps or go down a band size (from 38B to 36B, for example).*

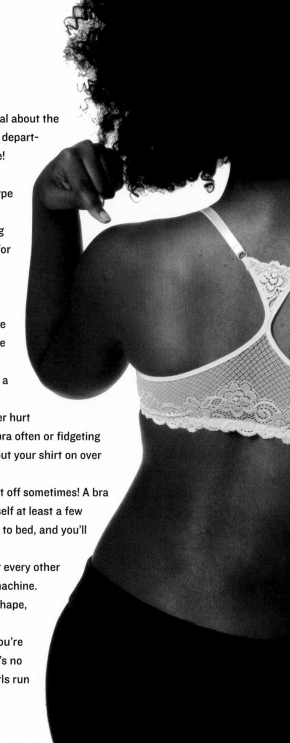

To avoid all these pitfalls and find your best-friend bras, be real about the situation. Measure yourself carefully (see page 97) or go to a department or specialty store and have a clerk measure you. It's free!

Picking the perfect bra involves testing many different styles and fabrics to get a perfect fit. The most comfortable type of bra is the cotton soft-cup, but bras with underwire provide more lift. When exercising or playing sports, consider buckling your breasts into a sports bra designed for athletic activities for even more support.

In your never-ending quest for a boob-worthy bra, you can also experiment with different features and ideas. Racer-back bras (at right) prevent falling straps and ease the pain of heavy breasts, while padded shoulder straps increase comfort. Also think about trying alternatives to bras: A well-made and supportive camisole might eliminate your need for a bra altogether.

Whatever you choose, remember that a bra should never hurt or feel uncomfortable. If you find yourself messing with your bra often or fidgeting with your chest, find a new bra. Before buying, make sure to put your shirt on over the new bra to see how it looks underneath your clothes.

Once you've found the perfect bra, don't forget to take it off sometimes! A bra is not meant to be worn 24/7. Try to hang loose and give yourself at least a few bra-free hours a day. At night, it's not necessary to wear a bra to bed, and you'll probably sleep better without one.

Bras should be washed after every use (or at least after every other use), either by hand or in the delicate cycle of your washing machine. Always let bras air dry, because dryers make them lose their shape, making you lose your money!

If you decide that no bra is the right one for you, and you're comfortable going completely without, that's fine, too. There's no medical reason you should wear one, so it's cool to let the girls run free!

My nipples are always flat
and never point out.

## WHAT'S GOING ON?

If your nipples turn out to be sunken treasures, you're one of at least 10 percent of us who have inverted nipples. Women with inverted nipples have a shorter than usual band of tissue that adheres the base of the nipple to the underlying breast tissue. The tissue draws in the nipple and creates an "innie." Sometimes only one nipple is inverted, or both can be.

To test your nips, gently squeeze your thumb and forefinger on the edge of your areola, pressing in toward the middle. If your nipple does not pop out or become erect after a moment or two, then you have a flat nipple. If it retracts or disappears, it's inverted. Flat and inverted nipples never protrude, even in the cold or when stimulated.

## HOW DO I DEAL?

There are no medical problems related to your nipples' shy behavior, so breathe a sigh of relief. If one nipple, however, suddenly decides to relocate indoors, *ask your doctor* to check out the change.

Even with truly flat nipples, a little bit of patience can sometimes coax your nipples out. The trick is to loosen the tissue that draws your nipples inward, keeping them inverted. One way to soften things up is a massage technique called the Hoffman, named for its inventor. Start performing the technique (see page 96) twice a day at first, working your way up to five times daily.

There's a surgical procedure that can correct an inverted nipple, but the complications include scarring and the potential loss of sensitivity. There's no medical reason to evert your nipples. When the time comes, most women with inverted nipples are able to breast-feed just fine, so don't fret about your future kid going hungry just yet.

Up to 10 percent of women have at least one inverted nipple.

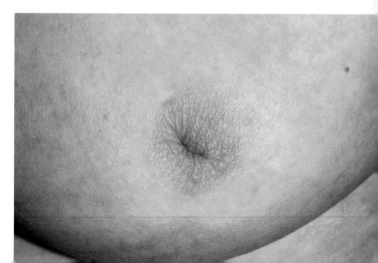

If you're thinking about taking Cleopatra's lead (page 83) and piercing your inverted or flat nipple, be cautious. While piercing can help to evert your inverted nipple, if the piercers don't know what they're doing, they could pierce your areola, creating numerous problems and pain. And if your nipple decides to re-retreat, there's a chance that the jewelry will try to go with it. Ouch!

## WHAT IF THEY NOTICE?

If someone notices your nipples and says something, don't get embarrassed. Be an extrovert about your inverted nipples! Tell them that 10 percent of people have inverted nipples, explain about the Hoffman technique (see left), and be proud of your uniqueness. Many people think inverted nipples are cool. Become one of them!

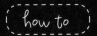

### DO THE HOFFMAN
#### (EVERT YOUR NIPPLES)

(1) To evert an inverted nipple, place your two thumbs opposite each other at the edge of your areola.

(2) Press into your chest firmly and at the same time pull your thumbs away from each other (toward your armpits).

(3) Repeat this step, rotating your thumbs in every direction possible: up, down, and sideways.

*WHAT YOU NEED:*

Flexible measuring tape • Mirror

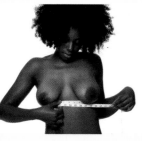

① Wrap the measuring tape all the way around your chest, right underneath your naked breasts (where your bra band will lie). Pull the tape as comfortably snug as you want your bra band to be. Take that number and add five inches to it for your BAND size. If the total is an odd number, round up to the next even number. For example, Marie's underbust measurement is 31, so when she adds five inches to that number, she realizes that her band size is a 36. If her underbust were 32 inches, she would round up her 37 inches (32 + 5) to an even bra size of 38.

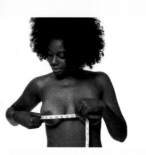

② Next, get your BUST measurement. Pull the tape up around the fullest part of your breasts (usually around the nipple). For the most accurate measurements, look in the mirror to make sure the tape is perfectly horizontal and try to keep your elbows close by your sides. Once Marie relaxes her other arm and looks straight into the mirror, her proper bust measurement is 39 inches.

③ To find out your cup size, subtract your band size (Marie's is 36) from your bust measurement (Marie's is 39) and then check the chart below. For Marie, the difference is three inches (39-36=3). Marie should wear a 36C bra.

*In most bras, as the band size increases, so does the cup size, meaning that the cup of a 34A is smaller than the cup of a 38A. As a 36C, Marie might fit a 38B or a 34D. She should try on several bras before buying one. In a comfortable, supportive bra, you should be able to fit one finger under the band easily.*

| DIFFERENCE BETWEEN BUST AND BAND SIZE | CORRESPONDING CUP SIZE |
|---|---|
| Less than One Inch | AA |
| 1 inch | A |
| 2 inches | B |
| 3 inches | C |
| 4 inches | D |
| 5 inches | DD (some companies call this an E) |
| 6 inches | DDD (some companies call this an F) |
| 7 inches | DDDD (some companies call this an G) |

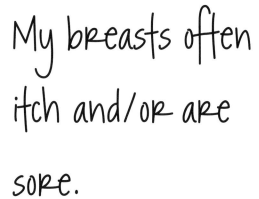

# My breasts often itch and/or are sore.

## WHAT'S GOING ON?

Your twin peaks might not have peaked yet! Breasts don't stop growing for years (if ever), and the growth can come in unexpected spurts. Making that much room isn't easy on your body, and the stretching of the skin around your breasts can cause itching and soreness.

Even if your breasts have stopped growing, raging hormones before and during menstrual periods can make breasts more tender to touch. Feel any lumps in your breast? If so, don't rule out the possibility of a harmless breast cyst, since a cyst can be accompanied by soreness (see page 105 for more information). Also, if your itchiness is accompanied by nipple discharge, or if you see darker spots appearing around or underneath your breast, you may have an infection, so be sure to *see your doctor.*

Another reason for itching or soreness may be that your breasts and nipples constantly rub against your clothing, causing chafing. Movement and moisture from athletic activities or sweating on your chest area can heighten the problem, especially in the warmer months. You may also have an allergic reaction to certain materials or be irritated by the soap you use to wash your bras.

## HOW DO I DEAL?

To soothe your tender ta-tas, try the cold compress tip in the sidebar. Take off your bra as often as you can to give your girls some breathing room.

Are you a new member of the boob-bearing club? If so, take comfort in the fact that this discomfort won't last long—probably less than a year. Eventually, the tenderness will decrease and the fruits of this labor will be well worth the discomfort.

If you're chafing, make sure to keep your breasts clean and dry, especially the skin underneath them. Wash your bras after every other use and, if you sweat in them, after each use. Turn to page 92 to learn how to find good bras that are soft, comfortable, and made of breathable fabric (cotton is usually best). Wait for the itching and soreness to stop before branching off to underwires and push-ups.

If the itching is only occasional, try to remember what bra you were wearing when the discomfort began. Stop wearing it and see what happens. You could be allergic to the fabric it's made from, or it could be a poor fit. Also, try switching your soap or laundry detergent to see if that's the culprit.

If you fear a cyst or infection, *see your doctor.* A physician can confirm the cyst (and perhaps drain it) or prescribe medication to make you itch-free!

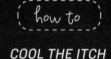

### COOL THE ITCH

For a quick pick-me-up, keep two bags of peas in the freezer. If your breasts become unbearably uncomfortable, lie down, put a towel over your breasts, and press the bags on top of the towel. The peas will conform around your boobs, soothing them and numbing the pain. Best of all, the peas are reusable—either as another compress or with dinner!

# BOOBY EMOTICONS

| | |
|---|---|
| (o)(o) | Breasts |
| ( + )( + ) | Fake Breasts |
| (@)(@) | Big Nipples |
| oo | A Cups |
| {O}{O} | D Cups |
| (oYo) | Wonderbra Breasts |
| ( ^ )( ^ ) | Cold Breasts |
| (Q)(O) | Pierced Breast |
| \o/\o/ | Grandma's Breasts |
| (%)(o) | Extra Nipple Breasts |

You can make these boobies with the keys on your computer!

# I have many little bumps around my nipple.

## WHAT'S GOING ON?

Know what those bumps are? They're actually Braille for "feel me." Okay, bad joke, couldn't resist. But really, everyone has a few bumps sprinkled around there. They're glands that secrete a tiny amount of lubricant to protect the nipple. In some women, these bumps are more prominent in size and color, and many girls even grow hair from them. (For more on this, see page 170.)

## HOW DO I DEAL?

Normal nipple bumps shouldn't change in appearance or be painful. If you find that one or more of your bumps has become more obvious or looks different, it could simply be that a hair follicle has become blocked with dead skin cells and oils, causing a zit of sorts. If a bump hurts, or if it is hard or swollen, *see your doctor* so you can be checked for infection. If the bump is not painful, keep the area as clean as possible and don't pop it; picking at the bump can cause infections and scarring. If you leave the bump alone, it will eventually go away, just as facial pimples do.

I have discharge coming from my nipples.

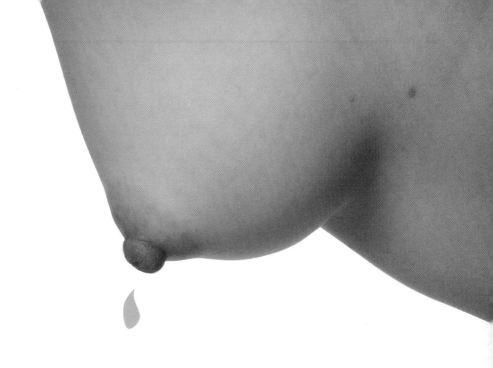

## WHAT'S GOING ON?

Although the very thought may seem gross (especially when it happens to you), brown, green, milky, sticky, or other types of goo may occasionally leak from your nipples for a variety of reasons. One possibility is pregnancy; when you are pregnant, your nipples can leak. It's also possible that you might have a hormonal imbalance. Are you taking any medications? Certain prescription drugs such as birth control pills and psychiatric medicines can cause nipple discharge in some people. In incredibly rare cases, nipple discharge can be a sign of breast cancer, especially if it is bloody.

## HOW DO I DEAL?

I know, it's really yucky, but infection of the breast and nipple CAN happen, especially if you ignore the advice on page 101 and pop a nipple pimple. If you start to drip from your nip, DO NOT SQUEEZE. Keep the nipple clean and dry, stop using lotions or perfume near the breast area, and _see your doctor immediately_. Reveal to the doctor all the gory details: color, consistency, and frequency of leakage. Chances are the discharge is not a big deal, but don't put this one off. See your doctor to clear up your mind (and hopefully your discharge).

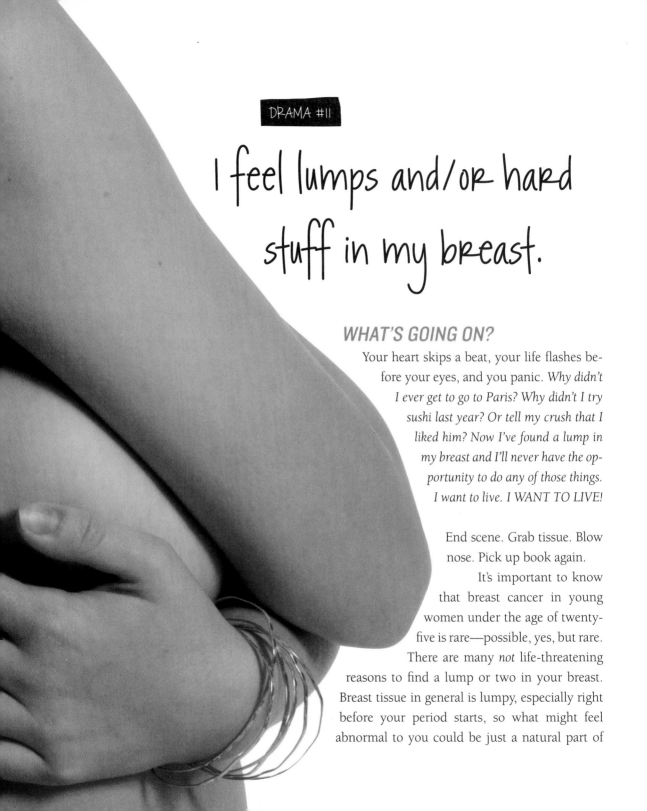

# I feel lumps and/or hard stuff in my breast.

## WHAT'S GOING ON?

Your heart skips a beat, your life flashes before your eyes, and you panic. *Why didn't I ever get to go to Paris? Why didn't I try sushi last year? Or tell my crush that I liked him? Now I've found a lump in my breast and I'll never have the opportunity to do any of those things. I want to live. I WANT TO LIVE!*

End scene. Grab tissue. Blow nose. Pick up book again.

It's important to know that breast cancer in young women under the age of twenty-five is rare—possible, yes, but rare. There are many *not* life-threatening reasons to find a lump or two in your breast. Breast tissue in general is lumpy, especially right before your period starts, so what might feel abnormal to you could be just a natural part of your boob makeup. Besides scratched pimples or love bites getting infected (yes, this happens!), three of the most common noncancerous issues that cause breast lumps are:

### FIBROCYSTIC (fie-broh-SIS-tik) BREASTS

This is a recurring (but harmless) condition of painful, lumpy breasts. More than half of all women have this condition at some time in life.

### FIBROADENOMAS (fie-broh-ad-en-OH-muhs)

Fibroadenomas are made up of solid tissue. They are not only harmless, but also painless, typically feeling hard and rubbery underneath the skin.

### FLUID-FILLED SACS CALLED CYSTS

These lumps may be the result of hormonal changes. Cysts are usually tender to touch, but while they may be painful (especially around your period), they're harmless.

## HOW DO I DEAL?

Wait until a week after your next period to give yourself a breast self-examination, or BSE for short. (See page 106 for instructions.) In the meantime, check your eating habits. Fatty foods and caffeine can aggravate the formation of breast lumps, so eliminating coffee, soda, and junk food might minimize the problem.

If the lump is still there when you recheck in a month, _see your doctor right away_, especially if it's hard or painful. While cysts and fibroadenomas are harmless, some studies show that they can be linked to breast cancer risk, and you don't want any bumps in the road to good health!

*fast fact*

*Why do guys have nipples but no obvious breasts? As embryos, both sexes start out with nipples and milk ducts. Both men and women are born with breast tissue, but testosterone (male hormone) stops the growth of breasts, while estrogen (female hormone) stimulates it. As time passes, women grow two perfectly working baby feeders, while most men end up with little leftovers. Because of the mother's estrogen, baby boys are sometimes born with small breasts, but once their own testosterone starts to pump, the breasts go away. Sometimes, around puberty, guys lose the hormone-balancing game, leading to gynecomastia (jin-i-koh-MAS-tee-uh), or male breasts. When hormones settle down after puberty, most male boobs go away by themselves, but some men grow such large breasts that they opt for reduction surgery to remove the extra tissue. See—guys have body drama, too!*

*Hello, breasts? Hi, how are you doing? Yeah, it's been a few months since I last checked you. I've been really busy, focusing on my other body dramas and—what? What do you mean, you feel neglected? I know we scheduled a monthly get-together, but to tell you the truth, I've just been so—huh? You want to show me a new bump that cropped up a couple of weeks ago? And a little mole on your side? Look, don't get upset. Okay, okay, I'll check you out. No, I promise I won't flake out next month, and if the same lump is there, we'll go to the doctor. Together. Because we're a team, OK? Hey, why don't we take some measurements from page 97 and I'll go out right now and get us a comfy new bra. Now are we even? Looks like it!*

In real life, it's up to you to maintain a healthy relationship with your breasts by giving yourself a breast self-examination once a month—no more, no less. Try to set aside ten minutes the week after the beginning of every period for this quick and potentially lifesaving test.

Don't blow off BSEs just because you're young. Although the chance of breast cancer under the age of twenty-five is small, keeping up-to-date with your boobs at an early age will give you a head start on knowing what feels right later. This is especially important if you have a history of breast cancer in your family. The more habitual you are about checking your breasts every month, the more easily you'll know if something feels wrong and the faster you can do something about it!

After completing the exam, if you find anything different two months in a row, *check with your doctor.* If you don't find anything, then take comfort in the fact that you've put your best breast forward!

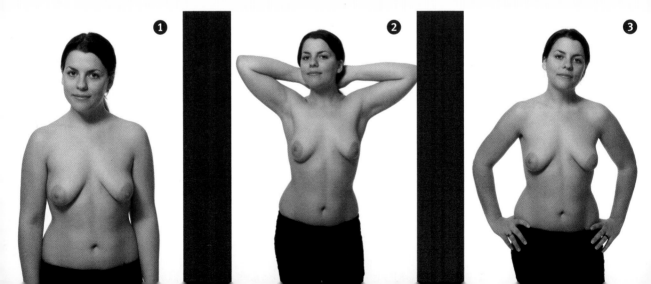

①  With your hands by your side, visually check your breasts in the mirror, looking them over very carefully. Do you see any changes in shape, size, or color since last month? Any new moles or freckles?

②  Place your hands behind your head and scrutinize again.

③  Place your hands on your hips and flex your chest muscles for one more gaze.

④  When you're in the shower or lying on your back (either way is fine), check your breasts by touch, using three techniques:

**Clock.** Making sure that the hand that isn't exploring stays behind your head, start underneath your armpit and move your fingers in small circles around your breast area, like a clock hand, working toward the nipple. Repeat for the other boob.

**Pizza.** This time, start from your nipple and move your fingers out toward the edge of the breast, dividing sections like a pizza pie.

**Sponge.** Next, slide your fingers up and down as if you're washing your breast with a sponge, covering the entire area.

⑤  Finally, gently squeeze your areola and nipples and look for any discharge.

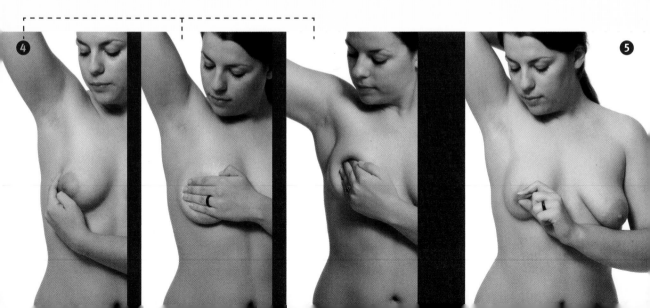

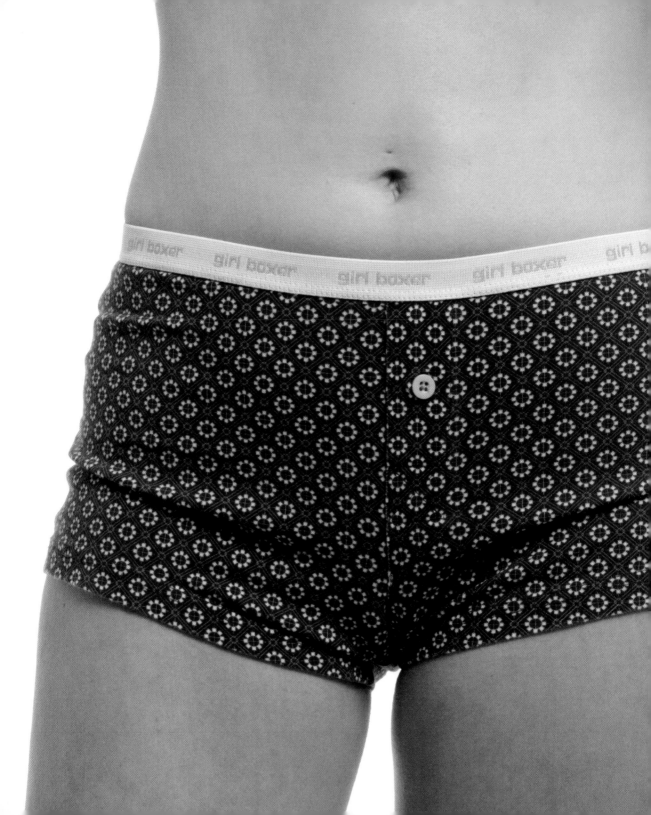

# DOWN THERE

NO. WAY.

Way.

YOU AREN'T!

I am.

IS THAT ALLOWED?

Why not?

IS YOURS IN THERE?

Maybe.

LET ME SEE!

Ok!

When describing this chapter and the accompanying photos to one of my best friends, that's exactly how the conversation went. I've known her for over ten years, but that was the first time we'd EVER talked about anything "down there." Even though we gossiped nonstop and stressed together about almost everything else, in the back of my mind, I felt that certain things I really wanted to ask about—like whether she thought her vulva was totally gross, too, or if she ever had problems going poo—were completely off-limits for discussion. For fear of embarrassment, I didn't get answers to the questions I had about my body until I started my women's studies classes in college, where anything was fair game. Until then, I thought that I was weird, stupid, and gross for even wondering. When my girlfriend excitedly flipped through this chapter and as we started chatting openly about some of our most personal concerns, I realized I wasn't alone in feeling silenced all these years!

fast facts

Society has brainwashed us! In a recent study by the Association of Reproductive Health Professionals, nine out of ten women said that they feel at least some shame when talking about their vaginas, and nearly 75 percent of us feel that talking about our vaginas has "shock value." DON'T become a statistic: Turn to page 116, grab a mirror, and get to know this very important part of you today!

Although we sometimes refer to our genitals as a vagina, that word describes only the birth canal, or the passage that runs from the outside to the uterus. The opening into the vagina, together with the external parts you can see, is called the vulva. It includes the inner and outer folds of skin, which are called the labia. Just in front of the vaginal opening is the sensitive part, the clitoris. The mound where your pubic hair grows is called the mons.

This is my favorite chapter because I think it's the one that can create the most change by combating a girl's worst enemy—shame. From fifth grade on, I always felt ashamed about my vagina and its surrounding parts. Was it too dark? Too deep? Not symmetrical enough? And don't get me started on my bowel issues! Having been brought up to think that girls should be dainty and pleasantly fragrant at all times, my frequent gas and horrible cramps really freaked me out.

We never look at other women and think, "Her skin isn't supposed to be that color," or "It's impossible for hair to have that texture," or "Feet aren't made in that size," because we've all seen thousands of different types of skin, hair, and feet, and we know that those body parts naturally and healthily come in countless colors, shapes, and sizes. Sadly, we don't enjoy such comfortable thoughts about one of the most personal and important parts of the body. But how could we? There's just not a lot of positive punani press out there. Cartoons portray us as having hairless slits, while pictures of most porn stars (the only other "real" bodies we get to see, even if by accident) are altered and airbrushed beyond reality. We're conditioned to think that things are supposed to look a certain way, so if our own equipment doesn't fit that close-minded bill, we feel as if something's wrong with us. Interestingly, most of us assume the worst without ever checking!

Studies show that fewer than 50 percent of women have ever given themselves a simple self-exam (see page 116 for more information).

Photographing fifty vulvas belonging to normal women between the ages of eighteen and sixty-five wasn't easy (go to www.nancyredd.com for the whole story), but it sure was a relief. I'll be the first to admit I was eager to peek. I was curious to see how my scrambled eggs compared with the bacon slabs of others. After the shoot, I certainly ended up with enough examples to compare and contrast!

If you're worried about what's up down there, look no further. In this chapter, for the first time ever, you'll find all the information you need to open your mind (and your eyes) about your most private of parts!

Once, the vagina was worshipped—literally! In ancient India, some Hindus were devout yoni worshippers, yoni being an ancient word for vagina. Ancient religious texts constantly refer to the yoni as the "divine passage," the birthplace that should be revered. Sounds good to me!

While guys continue to produce sperm throughout their lives, we are born with all the eggs we'll ever have. Although we only use about thirteen a year during our monthly cycles, we don't have an overstock of useful eggs. At birth, our ovaries contain well over a million eggs, but by puberty, only about 300,000 have not disintegrated or become infertile. The number of fertile eggs continues to shrink every year.

The average woman will have nearly five hundred periods in her lifetime and may use as many as 16,800 tampons.

# I hate the way I look down there.

## WHAT'S GOING ON?

What's up with those tiny, one-color, hairless slits that pornography suggests all adult women have? Sure, we look like that when we're babies, but as we get older, our labia lengthen and darken, our pubic hair gets thicker, and our clitorises grow, all because our body is proud to showcase its maturity. Adult magazines and videos choose to portray naked women as little girls down there, which is totally inaccurate, not to mention unfair!

It's hard to call our labia lovely when we don't have other normal, healthy woman-parts to compare ours to. Most of us only see our own, and when comparing ours to the digitally altered, barely there bits in the porn that pops up on our computer screens, our healthy, normal vulvas may seem strange in comparison!

## HOW DO I DEAL?

Worried that you're a disaster down there? Don't fret. The more familiar you are with each nook and cranny, the more beautiful you'll realize your uniqueness truly is.

Turn to page 116 to learn how to self-explore. Lock your bedroom door, grab a mirror, prop your legs up, poke around down there, and take a loooooong look. Now that you're more familiar with yourself, check out the healthy vulva spread (no pun intended) starting on page 118. Brace yourself beforehand, though. These photos probably aren't like any you've ever seen before, but chances are you'll find a vulva that looks a lot like yours. If not, that's ALSO a good thing! Each of us is one of a kind, and that's something to celebrate.

Surprised by how different the body parts in this book look from the ones you usually see in print? That's because we haven't done any fancy lighting tricks or retouching. These pictures are the real deal—100 percent natural—to give you the real facts!

## WHAT IF THEY NOTICE?

Don't forget, not everyone is as enlightened as you now are about how women's bodies are supposed to look. If other people are comparing your labia to the altered ones on their computer screen and in magazines, of course they will be confused. Try showing them this book, first flipping to the healthy vulva spread and then to "The Truth About Photos" (page 240) for an accurate anatomy lesson.

Also, many girls say rude things about other girls' bodies because they're not comfortable with their own, so do them a favor and show them this book, too. They'll probably be extremely relieved!

Bottom line about your bottom: If someone's telling you that you need to shave, that it's not supposed to look like that down there, or that you're smelly, gross, or weird, then he (or she!) doesn't deserve to be looking down there at all. You're much better off with someone who finds you beautiful just the way you are.

# LABIAPLASTY

Plastic surgery among young women is at an all-time high, and the latest, most disturbing trend is labiaplasty, in which a woman's labia is snipped to better resemble drawings and pornography of "ideal" women. Designer vaginas, as they're labeled, cost upwards of four thousand dollars and can take over three months to heal, but plastic surgeons' offices are packed, with some doctors performing forty to fifty labiaplasties a month on women as young as twenty years old. Even worse, this process of "perfecting" vaginas eliminates many of the most pleasurable parts! What's the point of having something pretty that doesn't feel good to touch?

F.Y.I.

Knowing about your body is important, and knowing exactly what you look like may be crucial to your health. When was the last time you took a good look at what's going on down there? There are many reasons to check yourself out: for health (to look for any changes or forgotten tampons), for pleasure (yay!), or simply for curiosity. By checking yourself out every month or so, you're getting to know a very important part of your body. After all, if you don't know what your body looks and smells like when it's healthy, how are you supposed to know when something's wrong?

Though at first it might be a bit difficult to see clearly down there, a brief peek is better than nothing. Start off by devoting at least two minutes to looking. Then work your way up until you can enjoy the view for as long as you please!

When's the best time? Whenever you want—hey, it's your body! You might not want to probe during your period for obvious reasons, but any time is perfectly OK and normal.

### WHAT YOU NEED:

Clean hands • 20 minutes of privacy (at least) • Bright light or flashlight • Large mirror (preferably a self-standing one) • Pillows and a towel

### WHAT TO DO:

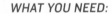

① Lock the door to prevent any unwanted interruptions. The last thing you need is your grandpa stepping in as you're shining a flashlight down there.

② Figure out where you're going to start. You could use your bed or lay a towel on the floor in front of a mirror. Prop yourself up with pillows so you'll be able to see the mirror reflection.

③ Remove your underwear, sit down, and bend your knees, keeping your feet hips-width apart and flat on the ground or bed.

④ Take a good look at the outside of your vulva. Find the outer "lips" (called labia) and spread them, revealing:

> • your inner labia (more liplike layers)
>
> • your clitoris (the hooded bump at the top of your labia that you'll probably want to pay more attention to later for pleasure purposes)

- your urethral opening (the small hole where your pee comes out)
- your vaginal opening (where the blood from your period is released and where babies come out)

⑤ Look down a bit and you'll see your anus. Notice how close it is to your vagina. That's why infection-causing bacteria can be so easily transmitted if you aren't careful to wipe front to back.

⑥ If you haven't been landscaping down there, you'll probably notice that there is a lot of hair, including around your anus. That's exactly as it should be.

⑦ Ready to go farther? Insert your pointer finger deep into your vagina and push up. Feel something smooth and firm, like the tip of your nose? That's your cervix you're touching! The cervix is the lower end of the uterus, which is where babies develop when a woman is pregnant.

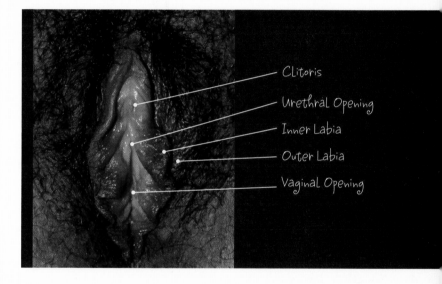

Clitoris
Urethral Opening
Inner Labia
Outer Labia
Vaginal Opening

⑧ OK, not to be gross, but you know you want to smell your finger. Go ahead. It's your body! Feel free to stay longer to sniff, poke, rub, or whatever feels good to you.

⑨ Once you've gotten an idea of the basic layout, you may want to backtrack to your clitoris. Just like a man's penis, it's full of nerve endings that are sensitive and pleasurable to touch. It deserves a thorough exploration!

*vagina,* that word only describes the birth canal, or the passage that runs from the outside to the uterus. The opening into the vagina, together with the external parts, is called the vulva, and that's what you see here.

OK, I'll admit that there's a pretty good reason why so many women haven't seen their own vulvas—it's extremely hard to get a good look, and even when we do, most of the time our view is upside down!

Figuring out how to photograph women "down there" was a challenge, to say the least, but my participants were total troupers who were more than pleased to drop trou in the name of eradicating vaginal shame. When I finally saw all of the vulvas in a row, I was overwhelmed with a variety of emotions—excitement, curiosity, and shock. At first, you might find this "spread" quite alien. After all, we're not used to looking at our OWN vagina, much less those of perfect strangers! But when I study the different vulvas, I see elements of my own here and there, and realize that no one's exactly the same. I also have been able to release a lot of the embarrassment I always carried around about my own vag. I hope that these pages will do the same for you!

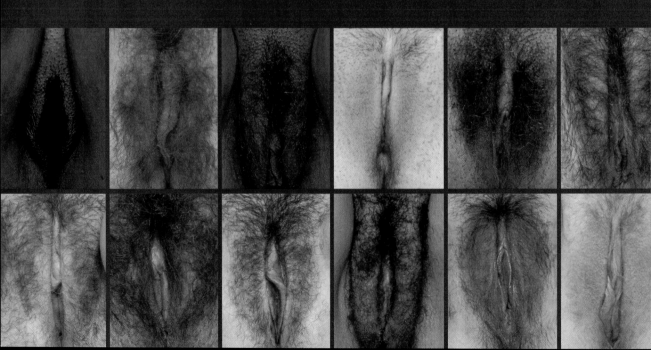

# 36 NICKNAMES FOR VULVAS

| | | |
|---|---|---|
| Beaver | Flower | Peach |
| Bird's Nest | Fur Burger | Poontang |
| Brillo Pad | Grassy Knoll | Pudenda |
| Bush | Honey Pot | Punani |
| Carpet | Hoo-ha | Quim |
| Cha-Cha | Jelly Roll | Rosebud |
| Chia Pet | Jewel Box | Rug |
| Cooter | Kitty Cat | Scrambled Eggs |
| Coochie | Minge | Trim |
| Crotch | Muff | Velcro Triangle |
| Curtains | Nappy Dugout | Vertical Smile |
| Flaming Lips | Pink Taco | The Wonder Down Under |

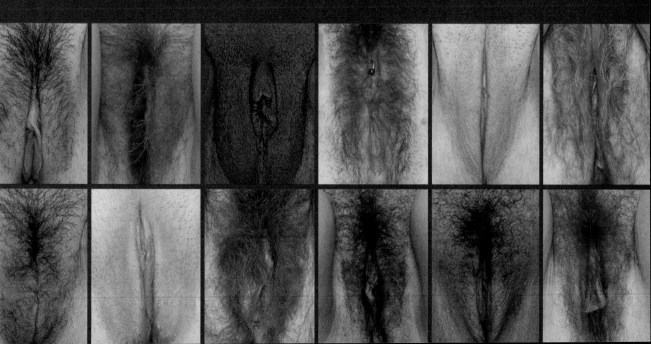

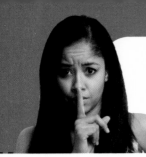

# i confess:
# i had a bump down there.

I felt it while shaving. The bump was large, hard, and slightly painful, and I was certain that it was cancer of the vulva or some awful, permanent disfigurement. It was the summer after my freshman year at Harvard, and I was back home in southern Virginia. The fact that I was hundreds of miles away from my faithful college doctor freaked me out. I had NO idea how to get help at home, and I couldn't imagine asking my mom! There was no way I could talk to her about it . . . what if she asked me about my personal life or something? I weighed the pros and cons: If I told my mom, I could figure out what the bump meant and how long I had to live. But if I told her, she might (OHMYGOODNESS) ask me if I was having SEX!

I decided to press my luck, and I waited an entire week for the bump to disappear on its own. Of course, it didn't. It actually got bigger! And more painful! I was a nervous wreck.

Finally, I caved. The next morning at breakfast, I blurted out, "Mom, I kinda don't feel good down there. Do you know a doctor or someone I could see?"

"Sure, darling, my gynecologist, the one who birthed you. I'll call and set up an appointment for tomorrow."

Great. I was about to be diagnosed with a deadly STI by the man who brought me into this world. Could it get any more embarrassing?

"Nancy, do you want me to come with you?"

"Mom, NO!"

The next day, in my crunchy paper gown, I nervously waited for the doctor and prepared for the worst.

"Hello, Miss Redd! To what do I owe this pleasure?"

I explained my bump, which, for some reason, already didn't seem as bad. The doctor was a really cool guy! He nodded and boomed, "Let me take a look-see!" In seconds, he was staring at my vulva. "Uh-huh, you've got an infected hair follicle down there! It happens when you shave sometimes." Before I could get too embarrassed, he quickly drained the pimple and told me I could put my skirt on. After asking me personal questions about my health history and whether my college doctor had given me a Pap test and pelvic exam in the last six months (which she had), he handed me a brown paper bag (which, when I opened, I found full of condoms), said good-bye, and scooted off to the next patient.

That was it?

That was it!

# It's bumpy and lumpy down there.

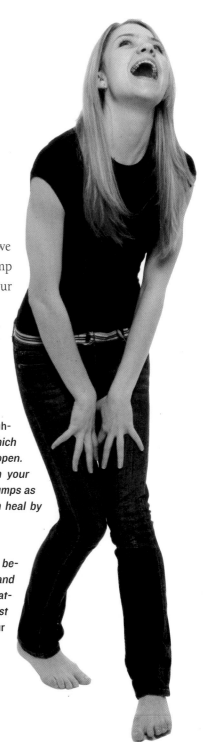

## WHAT'S GOING ON?

We're all afraid of things that go bump in the night, especially when we feel them in our crotches! First, know that the most prominent bump down there is the best one—your clitoris (see "How To: Explore Your Body" on page 116 for more information).

If your vulva has always had goose bumps in places, they're probably just part of your natural anatomy. However, if the landscape just recently turned into a rocky road, there are a few possible reasons:

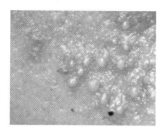

### INFECTED HAIR FOLLICLES

*Medically known as folliculitis (fuh-lick-yuh-LIE-tis). Hair follicles are the sacs from which hair grows and into which the oil glands open. They can become infected anywhere on your body, including down there. Treat these bumps as you would pimples: Do not pop. Let them heal by themselves.*

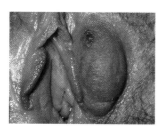

### BARTHOLIN'S DUCT CYSTS

*These happen when glands on your labia become blocked, creating round, hard, and sometimes painful bumps. Again, do not attempt to pop these cysts yourself. If the cyst continues to grow or is painful, see your doctor.*

(Turn to the next page for more bumps.)

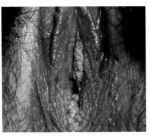

**GENITAL WARTS**

*These are sexually transmitted infections (STIs) caused by the human papilloma virus (HPV). Genital warts are painless. When visible, they look like tiny cauliflowers. Genital warts must be medically diagnosed and treated, so see your doctor.*

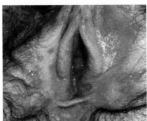

**GENITAL HERPES**

*This STI is caused by the herpes simplex virus 2 (HSV-2, see page 37 for more information). The virus causes painful blisters that can appear on the genital area, the skin around the anus, and sometimes on your face and mouth. This, too, requires a doctor's diagnosis and treatment.*

## HOW DO I DEAL?

*Never* pop vaginal bumps, because this impatient move can cause scarring and infection, not to mention a whole lot of pain. Ouch!

> *More often than not, ingrown hairs will go away by themselves, but after a week or so of careful observation, see your doctor if the bump*
> - is becoming larger, redder, more tender, or smellier, or
> - is accompanied by pain, itching, burning, or odor.

It's especially important to see your doctor if you're sexually active and the pimple persists. A lot of the time, a vulva bump is only an infected hair follicle. Sometimes, however, it's a much more serious issue, like genital warts or herpes. If it turns out to be an STI, your doctor can prescribe medication to keep your body as healthy as possible. While there is no cure for genital herpes, the faster you start medication, the better you'll be able to prevent outbreaks and complications. If you're worried, go ahead and make the appointment. Remember, *when in doubt, check it out!* Whether it's only a pimple or something more, you'll be better off in the end!

# HPV

Did you know that there is one sexually transmitted infection (STI) that over 80 percent of women get by the time they're fifty years old? It's the human papilloma virus, or HPV. When cauliflower-shaped warts are visible on the genitals, HPV can be diagnosed, and your doctor can apply medication to take away the visible lesions.

But not every type of HPV has visible signs or symptoms, making the infection hard to catch without your doctor specifically testing for it. Unlike women, men with HPV rarely show any signs of it, making it difficult to detect. Though about half of American men will have HPV at some point in their lives, only I percent of men have genital warts at any given time.

The HPV virus itself isn't yet curable, and it can pose a serious threat to your health. Sometimes it is associated with cervical cancer. Luckily, there's a new HPV vaccine that prevents HPV-associated cancers, as well as some strains of genital warts, and even common warts like the ones you find on your hands and feet. While it's considered best for very young girls (as young as nine) to get the vaccine before they become sexually active, all women under the age of twenty-six should receive the vaccine. The vaccine is given in the doctor's office in a series of three different shots strategically spaced a few months apart. It won't protect against ALL types of genital warts, but because there are no known side effects at present time, and also because many insurance companies and programs are administering the vaccine for no or low cost, the protection it offers is certainly worth looking into! Unfortunately, if you're already infected with a type of HPV that the vaccine protects against, you will not be cured by the vaccine, but you will be immunized from catching the other strands. Before giving you the vaccine, the doctor usually tests for HPV by checking your cervical cells, which makes it possible to find out if you have HPV even you aren't in the middle of an outbreak at the time.

*See your doctor* for more information on the vaccine or about testing for HPV.

DRAMA #3

# My vagina smells.

## WHAT'S GOING ON?

What did the blind man say as he passed the seafood market? "Hello, ladies!"

Jokes like that (though that one is kinda funny) make us clamp our legs in fear every time someone says the word *fish,* but in actuality, there is no such thing as a vagina that *doesn't* smell! Naturally, every woman's mix of hormones and diet produces unique discharges and distinctive scents from her vagina that can be musky, sweet, acidic . . . or a combination of all three. Few things are as frightening as fearing you've got crotch rot, but as author Eve Ensler says in *The Vagina Monologues,* it's not supposed to smell like rose petals!

Your vagina is, however, supposed to smell like YOU, and it's your responsibility to brave your bod often enough so you'll know whether there's a problem. See page 116 to start getting to know your vagina and your smells today.

Although girls often blame vaginal odor on yeast infections, it's rare that yeast infections smell. Yeast infections usually just itch a lot (see page 128 for more information). A common infection that is well-known for its funky odor is bacterial vaginosis, or BV for short. BV can occur for a variety of reasons; the exact cause isn't yet understood. Its awful odor is nearly always its only symptom, but it may be accompanied by a milky discharge. While BV doesn't itch, if you stand the stink for too long, BV can increase the risk of serious complications such as acquiring an STI or developing pelvic inflammatory disease (PID, see page 129) after surgery.

## HOW DO I DEAL?

If you're familiar with your usual aroma and you think it's altered for the worse, *see your doctor.* Your doctor can take a quick and painless swab from your cervix and the walls of your vagina, look at the cells through a microscope, and diagnose the actual problem. If it's BV, a prescription antibiotic can usually clear the air in no time. If the cause of your stink is more serious, your doctor will be able to address that situation as well.

## WHAT IF THEY NOTICE?

No matter how pungent you might feel, as long as you bathe properly, change your pad or tampon frequently if you're on your period, and wear clean clothes, your friends and the other people around you shouldn't be able to smell you—unless you've got an infection.

Concerned about intimate situations? A bathroom break gives you the opportunity to quickly wash your vulva. While douching is completely off-limits, a light spritz of fragrance on your inner thighs (but NOT on your sensitive parts) might make you more proud of your personal perfume.

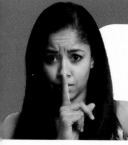

## i confess:
## i had bv while writing this book.

I still can't believe I'm admitting this. So I'm typing away, researching the symptoms of different types of vaginal infections that a woman might get . . . and I start to recognize myself in the text . . . and I immediately begin freaking out. For a couple of weeks, I'd noticed that my, ahem, eau de Nancy had not been up to its normal standard. I had blamed it on my diet, but after facing facts that it wasn't getting any better, I finally mustered up the courage to schedule an appointment with my doctor. "I think I have a vaginal infection" was all I had to say on the phone, and she made room for me in her packed schedule the very next day! Twenty-four hours later, I had an inexpensive prescription and a load off my shoulders. Sure enough, after a few days the air was clearer, my vagina fresher, and my book had already helped one person—me!

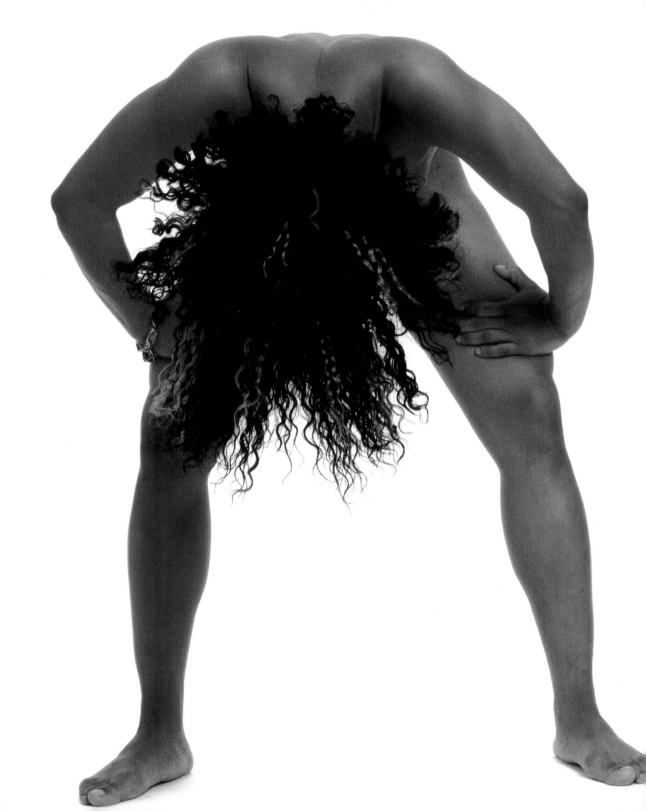

# My vagina secretes stuff.

## WHAT'S GOING ON?

Does it sometimes look as if somebody sneezed in your underwear?

In the same way that your eyes and nose drain mucus, so does your vagina—usually less than a teaspoon daily. Your vagina produces various types of discharge to keep itself moist, protect against infections, and wash out old cells in order to stay clean and healthy. As the month goes on, your vagina's pH balance changes at various times during your menstrual cycle. This causes the type and quantity of fluids your vagina secretes to change— the discharge varying in color, smell, and texture. Vaginal discharge is a perfectly normal bodily function, but certain discharges can signal that things down there are not in the pink.

*Any of the following symptoms warrants a visit to your doctor:*

- discharge that is an unusual color, such as yellow or green
- funky and foul odors
- a greater than usual quantity of discharge for an extended period of time
- anything painful or accompanied by sores

*fast fact*

*What was THAT? Have you ever, well, farted out of your vagina? Sometimes, during vigorous activity like bike riding, swimming, sex, or other exercising, your vagina takes in a lot of air and needs to burp it out. In doing so, it makes a flatulent noise that is called a queef. Queefing is odorless and painless, but it can be slightly ticklish (and extremely funny) when the air is released.*

A combination of any of those symptoms signifies one of these common vaginal infections, all of which can be medically treated:

### YEAST INFECTION

Everyone's vagina has a little bit of yeast, but when too much grows (a common occurrence), an itchy infection follows, medically known as candidiasis **(kan-dih-DIE-uh-sis)**. There is no serious smell associated with yeast infections, but common symptoms include white, clumpy discharge paired with itching, pain, and swelling of the vulva. Over-the-counter medicine or treatments prescribed by your doctor will usually clear the yeast infection in a week. You can prevent a yeast infection by immediately changing out of tight, wet clothing, such as workout gear or bathing suits, after you've finished using them.

### BACTERIAL VAGINOSIS

This "stinky" infection usually has few signs other than a pungent odor, but it may be paired with itching and redness in some cases. See page 124 for more information on BV.

### TRICHOMONIASIS (trik-uh-muh-NIE-uh-sis)

This sexually transmitted infection (STI) is associated with discharge that may be greenish or yellow in color, with a frothy or bubbly appearance. Yuk!

### CHLAMYDIA (kluh-MID-ee-uh) or GONORRHEA (gon-uh-REE-uh)

Most of the time the STIs chlamydia and gonorrhea have no symptoms and are not diagnosable without medical testing, but they sometimes are paired with vaginal discharge and a noticeable smell.


## HOW DO I DEAL?

If you're worried that you're dealing with dangerous discharge, a good way to keep tabs is to remember this rhyme: *If it's clear or white, it's all right. If it smells or it's itchy, something's fishy.*

Though over-the-counter treatments are available for itching and discomfort, *a visit to your doctor* is the best way to diagnose and treat your discharge. A doctor can tell you whether it's a yeast infection or an STI and can give you tips on how to avoid future occurrences.

Interested in knowing what discharge pattern is normal for you? Savvy women can know when their periods will begin simply by doing a quick finger check. Keep track each morning by gently inserting your pointer finger into your vagina and wiggling it around. After you pull your finger out, press it into your thumb, then slowly separate the two, checking to see what the discharge does.

*Here are some ways your discharge may appear:*
- When you're ovulating, a sticky, clear liquid usually appears in your underwear to signify that you're in your most fertile time.
- Right after your period, a brown, gummy discharge is normal (that's just old blood leaving your system).
- Other times, a watery, clear, odorless discharge is commonplace anytime during your cycle. It's part of your body's natural lubricant and is nothing to worry about.

Jot this information down and evaluate how your discharge changes throughout the month. To download your very own discharge calendar for keeping track, go to www.nancyredd.com.

If you're sexually active, don't rule out an STI. While the STIs mentioned above are completely curable, they can develop into more serious medical problems, such as pelvic inflammatory disease (PID), if left unchecked for too long. PID is the most common STI complication with the most serious effects, such as fertility problems, chronic pain, and other complications. Every year, more than 100,000 American women become infertile because of it, and more than a hundred women die from PID or its complications. Luckily, PID can be treated by a doctor, so don't delay in scheduling a checkup today!

# DON'T DOUCHE!

F.Y.I.

"To douche or not to douche?" That is a popular question, and the answer is NO! Douching is the act of washing your vagina with water or special cleansers that are often prepackaged in a squirt bottle for easy distribution of the liquid. Sounds great, right? Wrong. Your vagina is a self-cleaning organ, meaning that its natural discharge automatically removes whatever grunge finds its way in there. Douching strips away the "good" bacteria that your vagina needs to stay healthy. What's worse, douching can push an infection into your uterus, fallopian tubes, and ovaries. If you're worried about the way you smell, normal washing of your labia and other outer parts will keep you fresh. There's no need to do double duty internally!

# STIs

Did you know that one in three women will contract a sexually transmitted infection (STI) before the age of twenty-four? It's no exaggeration that if you're sexually active, STIs are a real possibility. Fifteen- to twenty-four-year-olds make up nearly half of new cases of STIs in the United States. Despite increased information about condom usage and safe sex, HIV, HPV, genital herpes, gonorrhea, and chlamydia are on the rise in America, with teen girls leading the way in infections.

Remember, sexual activity is NOT just vaginal or anal intercourse. You can get STIs from oral sex and, if your partner has an open sore on their mouth, you can get some types of STIs from kissing.

Curable STIs include chlamydia, gonorrhea, syphilis, trichomoniasis, and pubic lice. Some STIs are incurable, although their symptoms can be controlled with medication under a doctor's care. These include HPV, genital herpes, hepatitis C, and human immunodeficiency virus (HIV, the virus that causes AIDS). Another STI, hepatitis B, clears up on its own in 90 percent of cases, but 10 percent of hepatitis B infections are for life. Many STIs have similar symptoms (or none at all!), and only a doctor can identify which one you have.

*If you recognize any of the symptoms below, it's time to be tested:*
- a change in your vaginal discharge
- anal discharge (that's not poo)
- sores or rashes in or on your genitals or mouth
- vaginal burning, pain, or itching, either in general or when urinating

*While abstinence, of course, is the best bet for avoiding a nasty problem, keeping free of infections if you're having sex involves:*

**ALWAYS using condoms during vaginal or anal sex and dental dams or condoms during oral sex.** The trick to this very effective method is making sure you're using them correctly. Read the directions on the box and follow them to the letter. Don't count on your sexual partner to know how, and turn to page 145 for the proper way to put on a condom. Proper condom and dental dam usage is the number one way to prevent STIs. Sure, your partner might think sex feels better without protection, but put things in perspective: If sex with a condom feels bad, imagine how awful and unsexy being diagnosed with HIV would feel!

**Spotting the sores on your partner's face or genitals and steering clear.** Someone with open spots, sores, rashes, bumps, scabs, or anything bloody on the body might be showing signs of infection. Kissing, fondling, or exchanging fluids with that person might pass the problem along to you.

**Limiting your number of sex partners.** The more people you have oral, vaginal, or anal sex with, the greater your risk of acquiring an infection. Just because you like someone doesn't mean you have to go all the way (and then some), no matter how much you or your partner wants to. Another reason to limit the number of partners: You don't always have to have intercourse to become infected. Genital rubbing can pass on warts and herpes without penetration. If you're really attracted to a person, get tested together before taking things too far. Lots of couples are getting tested together nowadays!

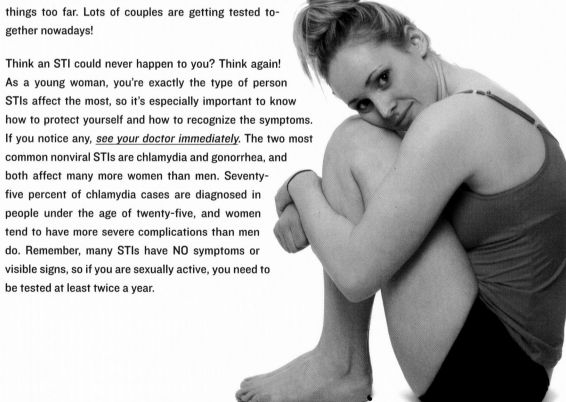

Think an STI could never happen to you? Think again! As a young woman, you're exactly the type of person STIs affect the most, so it's especially important to know how to protect yourself and how to recognize the symptoms. If you notice any, _see your doctor immediately_. The two most common nonviral STIs are chlamydia and gonorrhea, and both affect many more women than men. Seventy-five percent of chlamydia cases are diagnosed in people under the age of twenty-five, and women tend to have more severe complications than men do. Remember, many STIs have NO symptoms or visible signs, so if you are sexually active, you need to be tested at least twice a year.

Sometimes, you'll need to have questions answered or you'll want to obtain information and products without your friends or family knowing. Wanting privacy is understandable, but it's important that you get accurate information from people who know what they're talking about. The Internet and your best friend, while they may be great, do not count and are not safe sources for medical advice. Some of the "advice" found in chat rooms is downright dangerous!

If you have problems with your body, your family, your friends, or your significant other and want to talk to someone other than a doctor at a clinic, your school or college nurse can provide (or recommend) a confidential, safe space to find help. No matter how scared, embarrassed, or alone you may feel, there's always a place to go for help.

**Planned Parenthood.** If you want to test yourself for an STI or would like contraception, Planned Parenthood is a confidential resource to help you protect your body and put your mind at ease. Visit www.plannedparenthood.org or call 1-800-230-PLAN to find the center nearest you.

**National Family Planning & Reproductive Health Association.** Their Web site, www.nfprha.org, has an excellent "find a clinic" database.

**Phone Directories.** If you don't have a local Planned Parenthood, or if there isn't a clinic listed near you on the NFPRHA Web site, your area might have a community health center (like Dr. Diaz's Mount Sinai Adolescent Health Center in New York City), a teen program, or a family planning clinic where you can go confidentially. You'll find those places in the phone book or on sites like www.yellowpages.com. Check under "Health Centers" or "Health Services" in the yellow pages, or look under the government listing for your local health department.

**If at first you don't succeed . . .** If the first place you call can't help you, ask for a referral to the right place in your area. For example, I visited www .switchboard.org, an online national telephone directory, and typed "aids testing" in the business line and "columbus, ohio" in the location line. The first number that came up was not a local organization, but the second number that popped up was for Columbus Health Department HIV/AIDS Testing Site, and the person I spoke with was very helpful. It was that easy!

# 21 NICKNAMES FOR YOUR PERIOD

Aunt Flo Is in Town

I'm on the Rag

I'm at a Red Light

I'm Riding the Cotton Pony

I'm Surfing the Crimson Tide

I've Checked into the Red Roof Inn

I've Got the Curse of Dracula

I've Sprung a Leak

It's Leak Week

It's Red Cross Week

It's That Time of the Month

I Need One of Dracula's Tea Bags

My Dot

My Girlfriend

My Monthly Oil Change

My Red-headed Cousin

Old Faithful Is Spraying

The Curse

The Dam Has Burst

The Monthly Visitor

The Painters Are Dripping

Have some favorites that you don't see here? Come to www.nancyredd.com and share!

# My period is WAY too heavy or too long.

## WHAT'S GOING ON?

Sometimes Aunt Flo is uninvited and she RE-FUSES TO GO HOME. You may feel as if your menstrual flow is heavy enough to feed fifteen vampires, but most of the time, that heavy flow is just an illusion. In total, an entire period usually releases less than a half cup of blood, and that's including those gigantic clots that make you wonder if you're hemor-rhaging!

How can you know whether your period flow is normal? Heavy bleed-ing is defined as passing more than one cup of blood per cycle, soaking through a pad or tampon every hour for six hours in a row, or having a period that lasts more than seven days. If your flow isn't that large, fast, or long-lasting, then you probably just need to get used to the quantity your body naturally (and healthily) releases.

Some of us are heavy clot-ters, and we pass chunks of co-agulated (stuck together) blood during our periods. These clots come from uterine contractions and cramping (see the next drama for more information) so frequent that the blood doesn't have time to thin out before being passed. Again, a few dime-size or smaller clots a day during your period are normal.

## HOW DO I DEAL?

If your period truly is overflowing, you might have menorrhagia **(men-uh-RAY-jee-uh)**. It's a condition that occurs when the uterine lining builds up thicker and thicker, causing an extremely heavy period. It might have you not only checking the back of your pants often but also doubling over in pain. If you think you have menorrhagia or if you're passing a large number of extremely big clots during your period, *see your doctor* to make sure you don't have a thyroid problem or, if you're out of your teens, to make sure you aren't suffering from fibroids (growths on the uterus, a very common occurrence). Your doctor can prescribe medication or certain types of birth control to resolve the problem, relieve your pain, and lessen your monthly bleeding.

If you're just dealing with a normal, fairly heavy period, make sure to change your pad or tampon often to prevent smells and toxic shock syndrome (see below).

*fast facts*

*Four facts about tampons:*

① *A tampon will not act as a contraceptive, which means that it will not prevent you from getting pregnant if you keep it in during sex. (Ouch!)*

② *Using a tampon can't "devirginize" you.*

③ *Tampons don't make you bleed more than if you use a pad.*

④ *Tampons won't help you control urinary leaks. That's an entirely different hole! (Turn to page 116 to see for yourself.)*

# TOXIC SHOCK SYNDROME

F.Y.I.

Change is good, especially when you're talking tampons. Toxic shock syndrome (TSS) can happen when a woman leaves a tampon in too long or uses a tampon that is too absorbent for her level of flow. When too much blood collects in the tampon, for reasons that are not well understood, normally harmless bacteria release one or more toxins (poisons) into the bloodstream, making the woman extremely ill. Complications from TSS can even lead to death. To avoid TSS, change your tampon at least every four or five hours (and more frequently on heavy flow days), use the lowest absorbency possible, and don't use tampons all the time. If you forget to change your tampon, don't panic. Just change your tampon as soon as you realize the mistake and be on the lookout for flulike signs such as feeling faint, vomiting, diarrhea, or a fever. *See your doctor* as soon as symptoms begin or if you're really worried.

### MAKE AN EMERGENCY PAD

The tampon vending machine is out of order and there are no paper towels left in the dispenser. What's more, you used the emergency pad you carry in your purse when your period arrived early LAST month. The school nurse's office is closed and your girlfriends are as ill-prepared as you are. What to DO? Use these steps to fashion a sturdy, dependable pad that should at least get you through that second-period exam.

1. In the bathroom mirror, spot-check for telltale signs of your unexpected visitor. If some stains are showing, plan to tie a jacket or sweater around your waist until you can change clothes.

2. Find a stall with toilet paper (TP) and lock yourself in. Either sitting or standing, pull your underwear down to your knees and, using dry TP, blot the blood that's already made its debut.

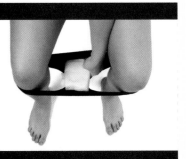

3. Wrap the end of the TP roll six or seven times around your hand until you feel the "pad" is thick enough. Remove your hand carefully and place this wad in your underwear, making sure to cover the part with the bloodstains, since it's obvious your period is flowing in that direction.

4. Remove a lengthy, intact piece of TP (about 10 squares) and place the end of it on top of the left side of your new pad. Wrap it underneath your underwear toward the right side, bringing it around and around until the paper ends.

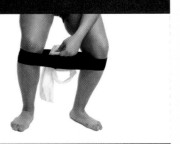

5. Repeat step 4 with another piece of paper. Feel free to wrap farther up to get more coverage and protection from shifting.

6. Carefully tuck the final end underneath, as you would a wrapped bandage, and pull your underwear up. Feel to make sure you've covered all potential leak opportunities. Then get dressed again.

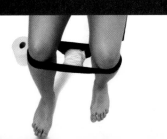

Voila! You've just saved yourself the worry of having a bloody piece of TP fall down your leg; this baby is immovable! There should be a Girl Scout badge awarded for this!

## GET OUT PERIOD STAINS

Period stains can be a bloody nightmare, but your favorite pants or panties don't have to look like a crime scene forever! Here's what to do:

① Run a sink or bucket full of ICE COLD water (hot water permanently sets bloodstains), and fully immerse the stain for at least ten minutes, preferably overnight.

② Next, treat the specific stains:

- For whites, dip a clean white cloth in hydrogen peroxide (available at any grocery or drugstore in brown bottles for under a buck) and gently rub the bloodstain. Peroxide has an amazing ability to lift bloodstains, but if that doesn't work, soak the item in a stronger solution of one part bleach mixed with six parts water for a couple of hours. Make sure you don't splash (bleach takes color out of clothes and carpets) and wash your hands immediately afterward.

- With colors, try making a solution of two parts water mixed with one part salt. Immerse the fabric, rubbing the stained area gently with salt to erase the stain.

③ After treating the spots, wash in cold water (never hot) and inspect before drying. If the stain is gone, feel free to pop the fabric in the dryer, but if it's still there, let it hang dry, because the heat of the dryer will set the stain. Repeat Steps I and 2 until you're stain-free.

If your underwear is the main clothing casualty, having a designated set of six or seven black cotton "period panties" is a good way to avoid this problem. You won't be able to see the stains!

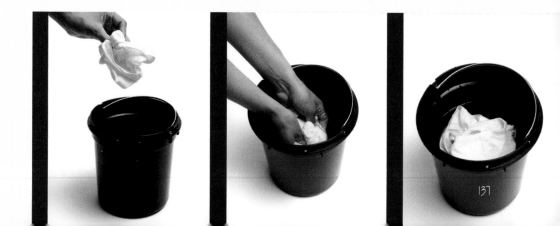

# I get REALLY bad cramps.

## WHAT'S GOING ON?

Period pains putting a cramp in your style? You're hardly alone! Eighty-one percent of women say they've experienced dysmenorrhea (dis-min-uh-REE-uh), which is the medical term for cramps, at some time in their lives. Cramps occur because hormones called prostaglandins cause contractions in your uterus by twisting the muscles down there, causing your abdomen to spasm.

The real function of prostaglandin-induced cramping is to help push a baby out of the uterus. However, for the 90+ percent of our lives that we're NOT pregnant and in labor, during the first few days of our period, prostaglandins cause nausea, headaches, back pains, and you guessed it—cramping.

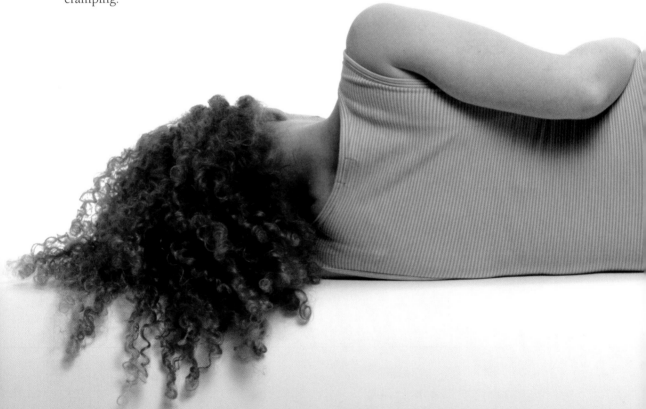

## HOW DO I DEAL?

Usually cramping begins a few days before your period starts and fades away after the second or third day of menstrual flow. Over-the-counter pain relieving pills can be helpful, especially if you start taking them as soon as you feel the first aches. Light exercises also lessen the intensity of cramping. A warm bath or a heating pad may reduce the pain.

While the first day or two of menstruation might throw you off your normal routine, the disruption shouldn't continue throughout your entire period. The phrase "No pain, no gain" might be a good mantra for athletes, but not for you when it comes to your period! If you find your period plagues are too problematic, *see your doctor.* He or she will check you for more serious problems that have cramping as a side effect. One common condition is endometriosis **(en-doh-me-tree-OH-sis)**, which is when extra uterine tissue starts to grow outside of the uterus, causing tremendous pain during your period. If your doctor diagnoses endometriosis or determines that your cramps are more serious than the average, you might leave with a prescription for hormones (such as "the Pill") to ease your pain.

*fast fact*

*Early lunar (moon-based) calendars were often based on the length of women's menstrual cycles, with thirteen twenty-eight-day months! It is thought that our cycles were once much more synchronized to the phases of the moon, but that connection faded with the introduction of artificial light. Still, our periods tend to be heavier, more painful, and longer in the colder months . . . so maybe there is something to the cosmic connection!*

# THE PILL

While the primary aim of birth control pills is to prevent pregnancy (see page 144), the hormones they contain serve many other purposes. Many doctors prescribe "the Pill" to women who aren't having sexual intercourse (as well as to those who are) because it provides a number of side benefits:

- **Lighter, more regular menstrual flow.** The Pill helps to keep your cycle predictable each month.
- **Less cramping.** Women are often prescribed the Pill to help with their period pain.
- **Reduced acne.** Certain types of the Pill can help clear pimply skin. Make sure you tell your doctor that you specifically want this feature, as not all pills have the same effect on your face.

Still, the Pill isn't perfect. Some side effects include spotting between periods, body sensitivities, headaches, and nausea. Also, you're ingesting extra hormones, so your emotions may fluctuate.

If you smoke, the Pill might cause life-threatening blood clots, so tell your doctor about your habits. Whatever effects the Pill has on your body, make sure to share them with your doctor. If you're using the Pill primarily for birth control and it's causing you problems, check out page 144 for information on other forms of contraception. You might need to switch kinds, or the Pill might not be the right choice for you.

## GIVING BLOAT THE BOOT

You know it's that time of the month when your favorite jeans won't button and you feel like a boat. Yep, you're bloated, and it's incredible how just a few ounces of extra water can make us feel (and look!) as if we've gained ten pounds. When you're trying to minimize the dreaded monthly spread, avoid consuming things that make you retain water, such as salty foods. Also, physical activity stimulates your body to release the water that's weighing you down, so try to exercise. Finally, constipation (the inability to poo) accompanies bloating, further puffing you up, so try to eat more fibrous foods (vegetables and whole grains) during your period.

# TAKING PMS SERIOUSLY

Premenstrual syndrome (PMS for short) used to be considered a figment of women's imaginations . . . as though we'd really cop an attitude and make up cravings for chocolate just because! Now we all know better, and we should take PMS seriously.

*The week or two before your period (and perhaps even right after it starts), do you notice*
- food cravings or an increased or decreased appetite?
- feelings of anxiety or depression?
- irritability or that you cry more easily?
- unexplained headaches or other body pains?
- bloating or changes in your bathroom habits?
- bigger and more sensitive boobs?
- fatigue that comes more quickly or more easily?

If so, these bodily changes aren't figments of your imagination. They're legitimate symptoms of PMS. The exact causes of PMS have yet to be pinpointed, but fluctuations in hormone levels definitely play a part in how we feel at different times in our menstrual cycles. PMS happens to all females: 85 percent of women deal with one or more PMS symptoms each month.

Just because PMS is a common concern doesn't mean we should resign ourselves to feeling bad for a significant portion of the month. There are many ways to beat PMS and to feel better emotionally and physically. PMS remedies include exercising to clear your mind, relieve stress, and get those natural painkilling endorphins flowing; getting lots of sleep to counteract fatigue; and eating a diet (or taking supplements) rich in folic acid (400 micrograms daily), calcium (1000–1300 milligrams daily), and Vitamin D (400 international units daily). Of course, doctor-prescribed and over-the-counter medicines are another option, especially for those who have more severe and longer-lasting symptoms. A rare few women have PMS symptoms so severe that they are unable to get out of the bed for a few days of each cycle. If you think you're in this category, *see your doctor.* Some extreme PMS-like symptoms can be signs of more serious illnesses. Your doctor can determine how best to help you. Different treatments work for different women. Although there is no cure for PMS, knowing what it is and when to expect it can help you to take control—and care—of your body and life.

# I'm a virgin, but I missed my period.

## WHAT'S GOING ON?

If you've never done "the do," but your period has said "toodle-oo," don't worry. Every girl misses a period or two at some time. If your period has just started in the last couple of years, it can take quite a while to get the cycle running smoothly, so be patient. Menstrual cycles rarely run like clockwork. Some months your flow may be heavy and last for a week, while other months you might drip for only a couple of days.

*fast fact*

*Tired of tampons and think pads are played out? From natural sea sponges (that you rinse, wring out, and reuse) to insertable plastic cups (that you pull out and empty from time to time), you'll find options and reviews at www.nancyredd .com. If you're not quite ready to make that jump, many mainstream stores are now carrying organic cotton tampons that are better for the earth—and, some studies suggest, for your body.*

Fluctuations are normal. Sometimes, an egg isn't produced, or there's just not enough uterine lining to shed. Most important, if a guy hasn't ejaculated near your vagina while you're making out, then NO, you are NOT pregnant. Seriously, you're not. There's no way! NO, swimming in the pool did not cause semen to enter your body. NO, you did not get pregnant from a toilet seat. Stop worrying!

If you are looking for a cause for your ceased period, ask yourself some questions: Have there been any changes in my day-to-day routine recently? Have I been exercising more or dieting too much? Have I lost a lot of weight? Am I under a lot of stress? Have I been traveling a lot? Any of these factors can affect your cycle, along with other internal issues.

## HOW DO I DEAL?

First, celebrate! You just got a free pass to skip a week of cramping and bleeding, and your absent friend will probably reappear next month (and you'll be wishing it would go away again).

If more than two menstrual cycles go by and you are still blood-free, *you MUST see your doctor.* You may have something called secondary amenorrhea (**ey-men-uh-REE-uh**), which is the lack of a period in a person who has previously been menstruating. While secondary amenorrhea itself isn't life-threatening, it may be a symptom of a more serious problem, such as low body weight or a hormonal imbalance. Your doctor will run tests to figure out exactly why your period has taken a break.

# WHAT IF I'M NOT A VIRGIN?

Ninety-five percent of Americans have sex before marriage, with 75 percent having sex before they're twenty. So, if you're sexually active, you're obviously not the only one. A load of responsibility goes along with having sex. You have to stay protected not only from pregnancy, but from diseases that could ruin (or end!) your life. Proper contraception (the medical term for birth control) is a must for anyone having sex, but along with figuring out the best type of birth control (which you'll find help with on the next page), ALL sexually active women should:

**Get the HPV vaccine.** The earlier you get it, the fewer strains of HPV you will have already been exposed to, making the vaccine more effective in preventing cervical cancer and some strains of genital and non-genital warts (for more HPV information, see page 123). Many clinics (especially on college campuses) offer the vaccine for free, so talk with your doctor.

**Have Pap and STI tests** so that your doctor (who will probably be your gynecologist) can check you for abnormalities and infections. Trust me, seeing the gyno isn't nearly as scary as thinking you have a disease (see page 120 for my story)! STI testing should be done *at least* twice a year. The only way to catch many STIs before they damage your body is by testing for them. Turn to page 132 for info on how to get reliable and confidential testing advice.

**Pay close attention to your period and discharge cycles.** Being sexually active means you're at risk not only for infections and disease, but also for unplanned pregnancy. By journaling your discharge and menstrual cycle (see page 129 for tips), you're more likely to catch concerns before they become too damaging or untreatable.

**Make sure that you're having sex for the right reasons.** Are you having sex because you feel pressured? Do you use sex to feel powerful or loved, to spite your parents, or to prove that you're grown? Are you practicing unsafe sex because you'd secretly like to have a baby, even though you know you might not be in the best life stage to take care of a child? If you answer "yes" to any of the questions above, talk to a nurse, counselor, doctor, or other trusted adult. Your body is special. Don't give yourself away or disrespect your body out of fear, shame, or loneliness!

**ALWAYS USE CONDOMS. ALWAYS.** Even if you're sexually active with only one person, and even if you're on another form of birth control, condoms are the best way to avoid being infected with an STI. Don't be so certain that your partner is telling all about their past sexual activity. People will say anything to get you in bed. Using condoms is a must for your health and your partner's. See the next page for directions on how to use them properly. Although condoms are an excellent form of protection, they AREN'T foolproof. You HAVE to use condoms (can I say that enough?), but you can't depend on them as your sole form of birth control.

# MORE ON
# CONTRACEPTION

Nearly 8 percent of teen girls aged fifteen to nineteen become pregnant each year. Sure, condoms are the most popular choice for contraception, but even when used correctly, their failure rate is about 2 to 15 percent. Of course, ALWAYS use condoms, to protect against STIs, but to be on the safe side for birth control purposes, always pair condom usage with one of the following contraception methods that you can get from your doctor:

## THE PATCH
Once a week, for three weeks out of the month, a square patch that looks like a Band-Aid is affixed to the arm, butt, or stomach. Hormones in the patch prevent pregnancy. Menstruation occurs during the fourth, patchless week. The patch failure rate when used perfectly is about 1 percent.

## THE RING
Once a month, a flexible vinyl ring is inserted into the vagina (it's unnoticeable once it's in correctly), where it stays for three weeks. After the ring is taken out, menstruation occurs during the fourth week. The failure rate for the ring when used perfectly is about 1 percent.

## THE SHOT
Every three months, the doctor injects a pregnancy-preventing hormone into the arm or butt. That's it! The failure rate for typical use of the shot is 3 percent (and less than 1 percent for "perfect"—correct and consistent—use). Periods usually become lighter when on the shot, and can stop completely.

## THE PILL
At the same time every day, a pill is taken that contains pregnancy-preventing hormones. In many types of birth control pills, the pill contains no hormones for one week out of the month, a change that induces menstruation. With perfect use, the failure rate for birth control pills is less than 1 percent. When pills are forgotten or taken late (this is considered "typical" use), that rate jumps to about 8 percent.

## DIAPHRAGMS, CERVICAL CAPS, AND CERVICAL SHIELDS
Diaphragms, cervical caps, and cervical shields, known as barrier methods, are smeared with spermicide (see below) and inserted into the vagina before intercourse. Barrier methods prevent pregnancy by blocking sperm from entering the cervix. Barrier method failure rates range from 6 to 16 percent.

## SPERMICIDES
These are creams, jellies, pellets, films, sponges, and foams that contain sperm-killing chemicals. They are inserted into the vagina before intercourse. Spermicides can be purchased without a prescription, and they are an excellent and easily obtainable addition to your birth control routine. However, they are NOT effective enough to use alone. Spermicide failure rates range from 6 to 32 percent.

## INTRAUTERINE DEVICES (IUDS)

An IUD is a plastic device that is implanted into your uterus to prevent pregnancy. It can be inserted or removed only by a doctor. If an STI or other infection is caught while a woman has an IUD, the infection can become more severe, causing sterility.

## FERTILITY AWARENESS-BASED METHODS (AKA RHYTHM METHOD)

Fertility awareness-based (FAB) methods include practices such as charting your discharge and carefully watching your cycle in order to tell when you're fertile. Needless to say, FAB methods are not effective (whose menstrual cycle or discharge schedule is always like clockwork?). You have other things to worry about, so stick with one of the prescriptions on the left.

## STERILIZATION

Sterilization occurs once a doctor "ties your tubes" by surgically closing off your fallopian tubes. This leaves eggs with no way of reaching the uterus, which makes it impossible for them to be fertilized by sperm. While this is a nearly foolproof method of preventing pregnancy, this option prevents any possibility of children in the future. Because of its irreversibility, it is only available to women over the age of twenty-one.

---

### EMERGENCY CONTRACEPTION

If you had sex without protection, or the protection you used failed (such as breaking a condom or forgetting to put in your diaphragm), emergency contraception, also known as the "morning-after" pill, can help you prevent pregnancy. Emergency contraceptive pills can be taken up to five days after unprotected sex, but the sooner they are taken, the more effective they are (if taken within 24 hours of unprotected sex they are, at best, only 85 to 90 percent effective). Remember, this option is ONLY for emergencies (hence the name) and should *not* be considered an everyday form of birth control. If you're in a pinch and need emergency contraception, *call your doctor or local Planned Parenthood IMMEDIATELY*. For faster service, be specific with your concern. Or, if you are over eighteen, you can obtain it without a prescription behind the counter from some pharmacies. It is kept behind the counter so you will have to request it and show identification before your purchase.

---

## PROPERLY USE A MALE CONDOM

① The penis should be erect before putting on the condom. Put the condom on before any contact is made between your body and the penis.

② Most condoms have a reservoir "tip" at the end where semen collects. If yours doesn't, pinch the tip to leave about a half-inch space while rolling the condom onto the penis.

③ Immediately after he ejaculates and before his penis becomes soft, he should withdraw, carefully holding the condom on his body with his hand to avoid semen spillage.

④ Remove the condom, wrap it in a tissue, and throw it in the trash. Don't try to flush it, as it may clog the toilet.

⑤ Use a new condom every time, and don't think that "double bagging" condoms equals twice the protection. It actually causes friction, which can cause tears in the material, enabling sperm and viruses to flow through.

# It hurts to pee and it feels as if I have to ALL the time.

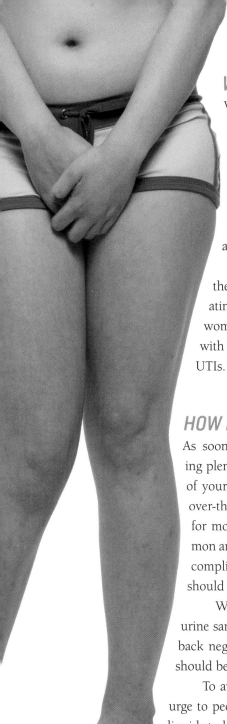

## WHAT'S GOING ON?

Without a second thought, we urinate about six to ten times a day, but when a urinary tract infection (UTI) occurs, this usually forgettable act becomes a true ordeal. When you have a UTI, the urge to pee is more frequent, and the urine comes out painfully and in small amounts. A UTI causes constant pressure or pain, in turn making you nauseated or giving you back pain, fever, or chills. Your painfully passed urine might have a cloudy or reddish appearance.

UTIs occur when certain types of bacteria find their way into the urethra or the bladder and multiply, creating a painful infection. About 20 percent of women have a UTI at some point in their lives, with some women having frequently recurring UTIs.

*fast fact*

*Certain foods and drinks can change your pee. For example, beets and blackberries might make your urine red, while asparagus can turn it green (and stinky) in some people.*

## HOW DO I DEAL?

As soon as UTI symptoms appear, start drinking plenty of fluids, especially cranberry juice, to help flush bacteria out of your urinary tract. To help with the pain and discomfort, there are over-the-counter medications you can take, but if your symptoms last for more than a day, _see your doctor immediately_. While UTIs are common and harmless if diagnosed and treated promptly, you don't want the complications, such as a kidney infection, that could arise if the infection should spread farther. Doctor-prescribed antibiotics can prevent this.

When you go in with a possible UTI, a doctor or nurse will take a urine sample from you. If you're sexually active and the urine test comes back negative for a UTI, tests for chlamydia, gonorrhea, and other STIs should be performed.

To avoid getting a UTI, make sure to urinate when you first get the urge to pee. Don't hold it in. Also, wipe front to back and drink plenty of liquids to keep your system flushed.

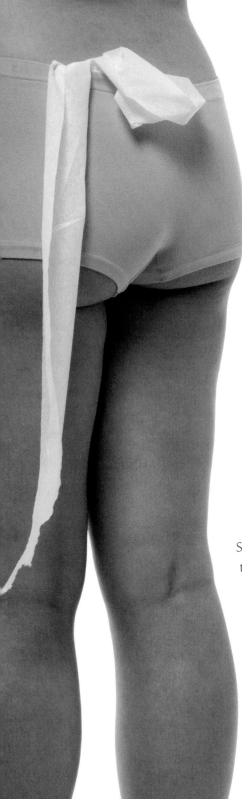

# I go poo too much or not enough.

## WHAT'S GOING ON?

Did you hear about the constipated math genius? She worked everything out with a pencil!

Defecation (the medical term for pooing) happens after your body finishes extracting all the nutrients it needs from the food you eat, and your bowels (intestines) literally move (hence the name bowel movement), making you poop.

*Some guidelines for a healthy bowel movement include:*

- **Color.** Most poos are some shade of yellow or brown.
- **Consistency.** Poo should be soft but have a shape. Many doctors say that a healthy poo looks like a sausage link. (Now, did that ruin your breakfast?)

Some people poo three times a day, while others get the urge only three times a week. Depending on what you eat, your poo can look and smell different every time.

If you find yourself "dropping the kids off at the pool" much more than usual, you might be suffering from diarrhea, which is watery, liquid, frequent poos. If you're going much less than usual, it's probably constipation, which is when your poo is dry, hard, and infrequent.

## HOW DO I DEAL?

From a bacterial or viral infection to disagreeable food to a reaction to certain medications, diarrhea has many sources and is a common occurrence. If you have diarrhea for only a day or two, remember to drink lots of fluids to replace the water you're losing. Dehydration is the number one complication from diarrhea. If you're still suffering after a couple of days, *see your doctor* because you may have a more serious problem (see the following page).

Lack of exercise, dehydration, and bad eating habits are the main causes of constipation, so to avoid being stopped up, try to stay active, eat at least twenty-five grams of fiber a day, and drink at least eight glasses of water. While poo-producing products such as chemical laxatives may seem like a good idea at first, use them only as a last resort, because overuse leads to your body depending upon the product to do number two.

You may need to take a fiber supplement to meet your daily requirements, but start incorporating some of these fabulously fibrous foods into your daily diet: oatmeal, apples, wheat bran, dried beans, nuts and seeds, citrus fruit, bananas, raisins, and more! Visit www.nancyredd.com for additional tips on how to improve your fiber intake.

Regardless of how often you go, it should NEVER hurt to go poo. Pushing too hard will eventually cause painful hemorrhoids or anal tears. Straining is a sign of constipation, so if "pinching a loaf" requires too much pressure, start drinking more water and eating more foods that are fibrous. Also, unless you've eaten extremely spicy food the night before, a burning sensation when you go is NOT normal and *should be discussed with your doctor ASAP.* Even when you're not feeling poorly, you should be checking out your poo.

*fast fact*

*Think your poo gets weird around your period? You're not imagining things, and it's not just you. During certain phases of their cycles, many women become constipated. Also, hormones (specifically progesterone and estrogen) fluctuate during your menstrual cycle. When you're having your period, hormonal changes tend to speed up your digestion, resulting in looser and more frequent bowel movements.*

*Danger signs in your stool include:*
- **Color.** Poo should *not* be extremely pale, black (unless you've taken Pepto-Bismol), or have blood in it.
- **Consistency.** Extremely runny or very hard, clumpy poo for an extended period of time is a sign of a problem.

*If you're noticing any of these irregularities, <u>see your doctor immediately</u>.*

Check out the follwing page for more poo problems and how to deal with them.

# COMMON
# POO
## PROBLEMS

Feel as if your problems are more serious than constipation or diarrhea? You might be dealing with a more complicated digestive problem in the form of celiac disease, irritable bowel syndrome (IBS), or inflammatory bowel disease (IBD).

### CELIAC DISEASE

This is an intestinal disorder involving an extreme sensitivity to gluten, a component of flour. More than 2 million Americans have celiac disease. When affected individuals eat cereal, starches, or anything made from rye, barley, or wheat, their stomachs become upset, causing constipation, diarrhea, bloating, cramping, nausea, and pain.

### IRRITABLE BOWEL SYNDROME (IBS)

This syndrome affects about 20 percent of all Americans, with the majority of victims being female. The nerves and muscles in the bowels of women with IBS do not function properly, causing sufferers frequent abdominal pain and unpredictable bowel habits. Constant diarrhea, recurrent constipation, or a mixture of both is not unusual for those with IBS, and certain foods make IBS worse. Only a doctor can verify that you have this condition.

### INFLAMMATORY BOWEL DISEASE (IBD)

IBD is a general term that describes conditions that cause inflammation in the intestines. One such disease is Crohn's disease. Another is ulcerative colitis. IBD has symptoms similar to those of IBS, but it can also cause weight loss, lack of appetite, and bleeding from the rectum. IBD can be associated with arthritis, osteoporosis, and other complications.

If you have any of the symptoms mentioned above, *see your doctor.* Your physician will run a few tests to diagnose and determine the severity of, and proper treatment for, your poo problems.

# WHEN IT HURTS TO GO POO

If you think the pain of constipation is as bad as it gets, you haven't ever experienced hemorrhoids (HEM-uh-roids). Hemorrhoids is the medical term for swollen, inflamed, and sometimes protruding veins inside your rectum or around your anus (fancy-speak for butt hole). About half of all men and women will have hemorrhoids by age fifty. Sometimes hemorrhoids just make you itch for a day or two, but hemorrhoids often cause tremendous pain—sometimes so powerful that the victim can't even sit down comfortably!

Many different things can cause hemorrhoids. Constipation with excessive straining or diarrhea with too-frequent poos can bring 'em on, as can sitting too much. Anal sex also causes hemorrhoids.

Sometimes you can see them, and sometimes they're inside of you. Wherever they are, their symptoms are hard to miss:

- Pain around your anus and inside your rectum. This pain may increase when you go to the bathroom.

- Bright red blood on your poop or toilet paper. Yes, you have to look.

- Anal itching from draining mucus. Yuk!

- Lumps (or a lump) around your anus. It's not uncommon to have no visible signs of a hemorrhoid, so if you notice other signs but are lacking a lump, you should still see your doctor.

*So what should YOU do if it hurts to go poo?*

- Drink lots of water and eat lots of fiber (see page 149). Soft, well-formed stool hurts less to pass.

- To avoid additional irritation from perfumes and dyes, use only white, fragrance-free toilet paper and wear only breathable, white cotton panties (see page 155).

- Take warm baths. Sitting in warm water can do wonders for your bottom.

- Most importantly, *see your doctor,* especially if you are bleeding. Sometimes hemorrhoid symptoms are actually signs of another illness, and on rare occasions hemorrhoids won't go away without a doctor's intervention. So don't stay quiet about your tush troubles!

# BOOTY EMOTICONS

| | |
|---|---|
| (_!_) | a regular butt |
| (!) | a tiny butt |
| ( Y ) | a perky butt |
| (__!__) | a BIG butt |
| (_._) | a flat butt |
| (_$_) | Money is coming out of her butt! |
| (_E=mc2_) | such a smart butt |

You can make these booties with the keys on your computer!

# I get skid marks in my underwear.

## WHAT'S GOING ON?

It's hard to feel like you're #1 when you're plagued by the unwanted presence of #2! Skid marks can be an embarrassing ~~pain~~ stain in your rear, and they mainly happen for one of two reasons:

① Farting where your expulsion of gas is powerful enough to push poo particles out onto your panties.

② You're not wiping properly after using the bathroom, leaving rings around your rump that ultimately end up on your underwear.

## HOW DO I DEAL?

Tired of your tail leaving a poo trail? You can't predict when you'll pass a butt bomb, but the easiest way to stop streaking is by working on your wiping technique.

For starters, use a new piece of paper after every wipe. No double dipping or you're defeating your efforts. Push up closely against your skin as you wipe, and ALWAYS WIPE FRONT TO BACK. ALWAYS. That's the best way to clean the area, and wiping the other way might actually push anal bacteria into your urethra or vaginal area, causing an infection.

*fast fact*

*Excuse YOU! Or was that me? Since it's normal to pass gas fourteen times daily, it's pretty easy to lose track! Anyway, she who smelt it, dealt it.*

There is no magic number of wipes. Sometimes one or two do the trick, and other times even three, four, or more aren't enough. If after a couple of wipes, the paper still won't come clean, dampen a bit of paper with water from the sink or use baby wipes. They work just as well as the "feminine wipes" you buy on the personal hygiene aisle, and they are much cheaper. Take your time, follow the above tips, and keep at it until the paper wipes clean.

## WHAT IF THEY NOTICE?

If you're skidding fairly often, wearing darker-colored, patterned underwear (as opposed to solid white or cream) can help to mask the marks.

**F.Y.I.**

# POO DEODORIZERS

Sometimes, even if you're not at the best place to do #2 . . . when you've gotta go . . . you've gotta go! It's bad enough if you're at your grandma's house (does she HAVE to ask you where you're going?), but what if you feel the need to drop the deed in the company of your crush? The very thought of a family member or friend walking in behind you to sniff your stuff is mortifying. That's why, recently, entrepreneurs have come up with powerful toilet bowl deodorizers that come in little dropper bottles. To have a scent-free poo, all you have to do is squeeze a bit of the liquid into the toilet bowl before you sit down. Perfumed oil will glaze the water, trapping the smell of whatever drops beneath its fragrant, hard-to-permeate barrier! (One product's catch slogan: Add the drops and the smell stops!) For best results, flush once as soon as you go, even before you wipe. Our test results found that going FAST (and flushing quickly) helps tremendously, along with using an extra after-drop for added security. Most importantly, if you've gotta pass gas, try to do a SBD (silent but deadly) BEFORE entering the bathroom. The drops can only mask odors of things that plop in the pot BEFORE the smell hits the air—and gas is all air, baby. For reviews on the best and worst stealth-stool products, check out www.nancyredd.com.

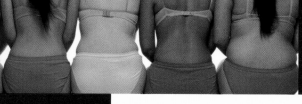

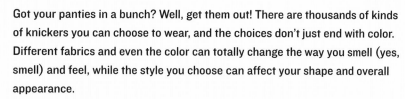
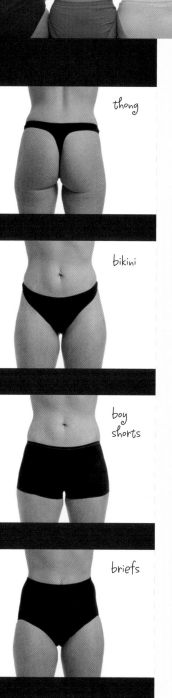

thong

bikini

boy shorts

briefs

Got your panties in a bunch? Well, get them out! There are thousands of kinds of knickers you can choose to wear, and the choices don't just end with color. Different fabrics and even the color can totally change the way you smell (yes, smell) and feel, while the style you choose can affect your shape and overall appearance.

**Fit.** The incorrect size or style can leave you with yucky pantylines and cause butt burn. Underwear that is too tight can pinch at your waist, crotch, thighs, and (in the case of thongs) between your cheeks, leaving marks, causing rashes, and making you itch. If your waistband is cutting into your flesh, size up. If there's extra fabric wrinkling around, size down.

**Fabric.** While silks, satins, and even polyester are fun fanny fabrics, they don't allow your skin to breathe, and they tend to trap odor-causing bacteria. Stick with cotton, or at least make sure your underwear has a cotton crotch lining. Another natural fiber bonus: Cotton and cotton blends also keep your body cooler, causing your pubic area to sweat (and smell) less.

**Color.** Covered in cotton and still having a crotch crisis? The dye in the fabric might be causing you to smell or scratch. When it comes to healthy undergarments, white is always right; but if you choose to wear color, make sure to wash all new pieces before you wear them to remove extra dye that may be irritating.

**Go Without.** There's nothing wrong with not wearing underwear whenever you feel like it. OK, perhaps it's not such a great idea to bare it all while wearing a miniskirt, but going commando poses absolutely NO health risks, and a breather can be good for your vagina, especially while sleeping.

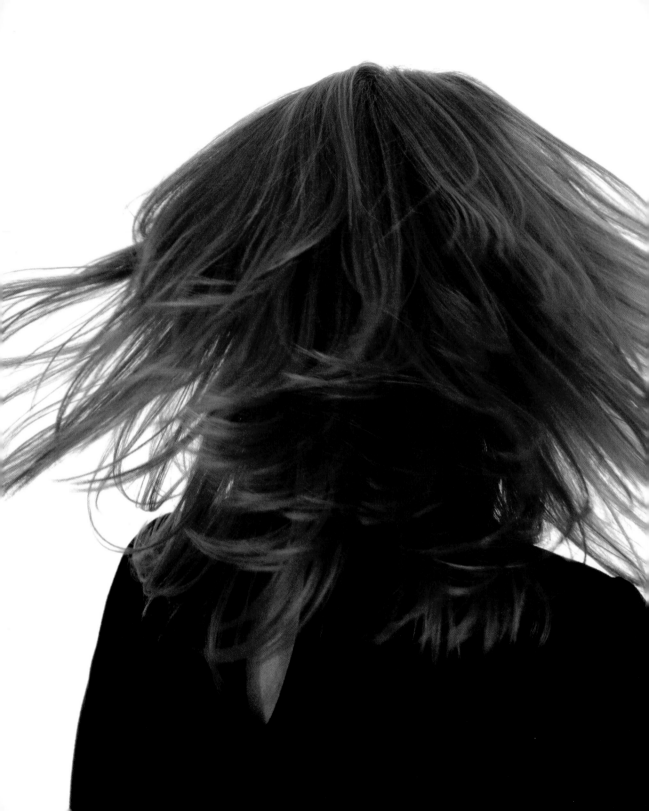

# HAIR
# NAILS
## MOUTH

"WHY ME!" I screamed, staring through sobs at my tress-filled hand. That weekend, my high school was throwing a huge party for graduating seniors. I wanted to look my best, so instead of waiting the recommended eight weeks between processes, I persuaded my reluctant stylist to chemically straighten my hair only a month after my previous treatment. The result? Clumps of hair coming out in my comb! I might have been able to convince my stylist, but no amount of pleading was going to keep my hair on my head. In a matter of days, I went from having a head full of beautiful hair to near bald. Because of my impatience, I had to cut off all of my damaged hair. I was about to start my freshman year in college, and I had NO idea how to style the natural curls that began to grow in. Needless to say, I was devastated, and the road to hair recovery didn't become any easier. It took weeks of tears, months of wearing nothing but ponytails, and many, many years before my hair grew back to its original length. Once it came back, I vowed never to touch hair chemicals again!

I'm not the only one who has learned about hair the hard way. I've learned some lessons about my mouth and nails, too. I have suffered from halitosis (bad breath) from forgetting to brush and from toenail fungus from hiking in soaked sneakers. Admittedly, making decisions about these things isn't always easy, and although my mind tells me that—as a strong, empowered woman—I shouldn't care so much about stuff like how my hair, mouth, and nails look, I can't help constantly painting and polishing all three. Sometimes, however, too much attention can have the opposite effect, and not just with hair. Incorrect care or overprocessing can also ruin nails and teeth.

Deciding what, where, and how much of your body to style can be a true nail-biter. No matter what you choose to do (or not do), it's important to remember that body beauty isn't just skin deep. The condition of your hair, nails, and mouth often reflects what's going on with your health. Every girl deserves an outer appearance that reflects her inner glow, so from bad breath to hair breakage, this chapter will help you avoid some major pitfalls—and not just when shaving your pits!

# It's a forest down there.

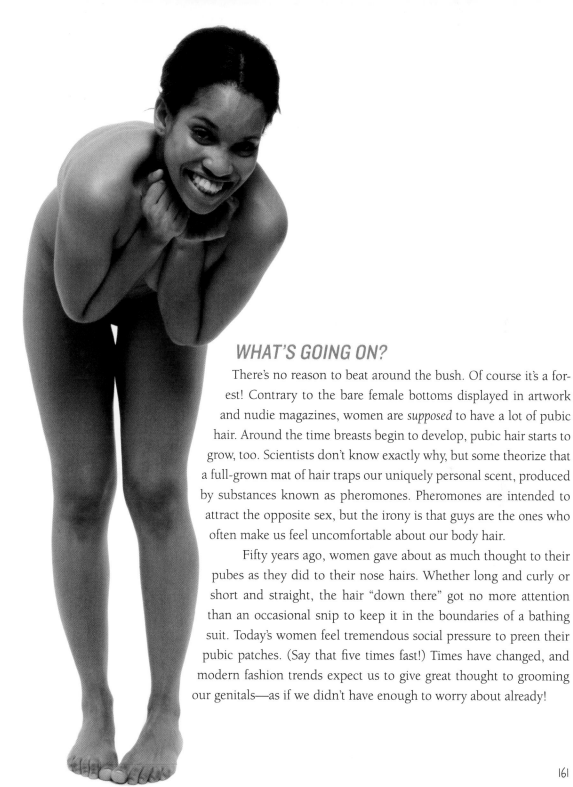

## WHAT'S GOING ON?

There's no reason to beat around the bush. Of course it's a forest! Contrary to the bare female bottoms displayed in artwork and nudie magazines, women are *supposed* to have a lot of pubic hair. Around the time breasts begin to develop, pubic hair starts to grow, too. Scientists don't know exactly why, but some theorize that a full-grown mat of hair traps our uniquely personal scent, produced by substances known as pheromones. Pheromones are intended to attract the opposite sex, but the irony is that guys are the ones who often make us feel uncomfortable about our body hair.

Fifty years ago, women gave about as much thought to their pubes as they did to their nose hairs. Whether long and curly or short and straight, the hair "down there" got no more attention than an occasional snip to keep it in the boundaries of a bathing suit. Today's women feel tremendous social pressure to preen their pubic patches. (Say that five times fast!) Times have changed, and modern fashion trends expect us to give great thought to grooming our genitals—as if we didn't have enough to worry about already!

## HOW DO I DEAL?

The decision to landscape your labia is an extremely personal one. Some people feel that removing pubic hair helps them feel fresher between showers, while others find it another interesting way to make a statement about themselves. Perhaps you can't understand all the fuss and have absolutely no interest in crotch coiffing, or you may want a haircut down south, but the hassle and upkeep (not to mention the itch of the returning hairs) are a turnoff for you. The choice is yours and only yours to make, so be sure that YOU choose your pube-do.

Curious about what you look like underneath all that hair? A good first step is to *carefully* trim your bush with a pair of clean scissors. Take extra caution around the most sensitive areas! Make disposal easy by trimming on the toilet or while sitting on a towel, and don't forget to wash the scissors thoroughly before use and again before putting them back in the drawer. No one wants to discover a stray pube!

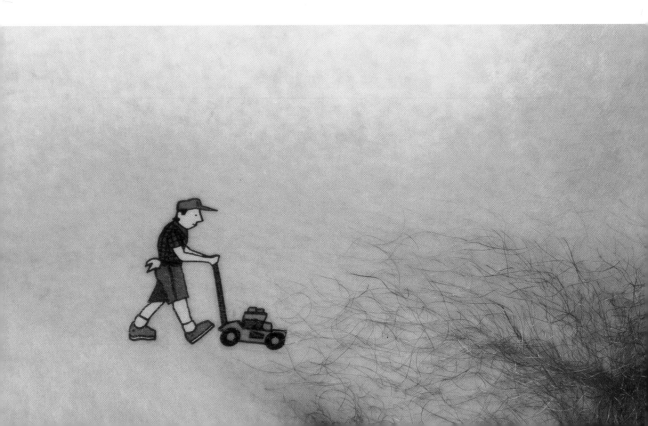

Next, you might experiment with removing hair, either carefully with a razor (tips are on page 166) or by getting a bikini wax in a salon (see page 176 for how to choose a clean and safe place). As with shaving your legs, ingrown hairs and razor burn are always possible (see the next drama for information), so be gentle and patient. Shaving in the direction the hair grows is safest.

Disappointed in your landscaped look? Don't worry, your pubic garden will quickly sprout up anew, giving you back your natural style in no time!

## WHAT IF THEY NOTICE?

If someone says something about your fluffy muff that makes you feel uncomfortable, suggest that your critic make an appointment for waxing so they can see how it feels. Tell faultfinders that if they survive it, then (and only then) you might consider a wax job, too!

# PUBE-DOS

In some cultures, pubic hair styling isn't just a personal preference; the way people wear their hair down there is mandated by society! Allegedly, in certain African tribes where nudity is the norm, married women must shave or even braid their pubic hair in specific styles to communicate their taken status. Don't think that women are the only ones with rules attached to their pubes. For many Muslims the removal of all pubic hair by both male and female adults is an important religious tradition. Don't believe that there could be even more restrictive pubic rules? Believe it. Until recently, it was illegal for Japanese drawings to show pubic hair at all!

People today remove their pubes on purpose, but in the seventeenth century, a heap of hair down there was a sign of great health. Due to sexually transmitted infections (STIs), vermin, and medications taken for these and other problems, many people lost not only the hair on their heads, but also the hair on their genitals. Bald-bottomed individuals who wanted to veil their venereal diseases (and who had money to spare) had wigs called merkins custom-made to cover their genitals!

My legs
feel like

chicken skin

after I

shave.

## WHAT'S GOING ON?

In your attempts to smooth things out, is your skin giving you a rough time? Hair removal can be hard on your skin. Professionals have many ways to defuzz our delicate bodies, but the easiest (and cheapest) at-home technique is shaving. Done impatiently or incorrectly, however, the process is dehydrating and can do a lot of damage, creating that "chicken skin" look and feel.

When you shave carelessly, you scrape the razor over the same surfaces repeatedly, causing hundreds of tiny cuts that might be too small to see, but that leave skin dull, rough, and lifeless. Sometimes, these tiny nicks become aggravated, either because there are a lot of them or because skin care products irritate them—as might happen if you use a body scrub on newly shaved legs. What you get for your efforts is a red, rashlike razor burn!

Razor burn isn't the only cause of chicken skin legs. Shaving often leaves behind blunt, flat-topped hairs that you can feel when you rub your hand up and down your legs. As these cropped hairs begin to regrow, their bluntness sometimes causes them to curl back into their follicles, causing large, painful bumps called ingrown hairs. Some people are more prone to razor burn and ingrown hairs than others, especially those who have curlier, coarser hair, but poor shaving preparation and techniques can create these issues in anyone.

Razor burn and ingrown hairs can also be paired with folliculitis (fuh-lick-yuh-LIE-tis), which is inflammation of hair follicles caused by friction and irritation (like poor shaving technique), resulting in tiny, pimplelike bumps on your skin.

## HOW DO I DEAL?

Do you feel as if you could grate cheese on your skin? The first step in putting the fire out on your legs, armpits, or bikini area is to stop feeding the flames! Give your skin a break and stop all hair removal for at least a week (preferably two) to let your follicles heal.

After your skin mends, start perfecting the art of hair removal. Check out the next page for some tips and tricks to help give you the smoothness you desire, while avoiding everything from ingrown hairs to major itching.

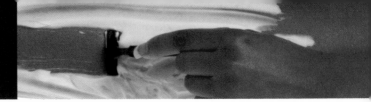

### THE PREP WORK

**A fresh, new razor** is crucial for avoiding nicks, especially if you have sensitive or bump-prone skin. Most blades, especially disposable ones, have only two or three shaves in them. Don't try to stretch the razor for more or you'll be flipping to page 137 for tips on how to get bloodstains out of your clothes!

**For best results, shave in the afternoon or at night.** Skin is slightly swollen when you first wake up, making it harder to get a close cut.

**Shave only in or after a shower or bath.** Warm water opens your pores, softens the hair, and helps the razor glide over your skin.

**Exfoliating beforehand** with a loofah or body scrub makes a close shave easier by removing dead skin cells that surround your hairs. This is strictly a "before" activity, as scrubbing afterward will leave you with irritated skin.

### THE SHAVING TECHNIQUE

① **Lather up (maybe).** Shaving cream can soften hairs, but it's messy to use. To minimize the mess, apply a quarter-inch thick layer only to the small area you're about to shave, reapplying as you work. For some people, regular soap or hair conditioner (which serves the same hair-softening purpose) works better than shaving cream, but depending on how your skin reacts, you might choose to skip this step. Some women fare better with just plain water.

② **Choose direction.** Rub your hand down your legs toward your ankle and then up toward your knee. The way that felt prickly is the direction you would shave to achieve the closest shave and cleanest look. Some parts, such as your underarms and bikini area, have hair that grows in different directions. For best results in these places, gently shave up, down, and then, if necessary, across. If you're prone to razor burn and ingrown hairs, shave WITH the direction of the hair, being very gentle with the razor and using as few strokes as possible to avoid irritation. While your shave might not be as close as it would be if you went against the grain, you'll still appear smooth and stay bump-free. This is especially important when shaving your bikini area.

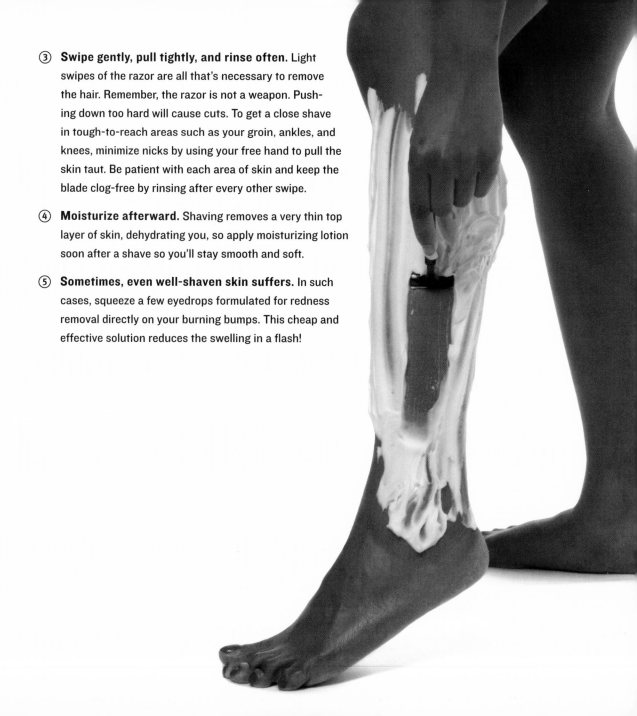

③ **Swipe gently, pull tightly, and rinse often.** Light swipes of the razor are all that's necessary to remove the hair. Remember, the razor is not a weapon. Pushing down too hard will cause cuts. To get a close shave in tough-to-reach areas such as your groin, ankles, and knees, minimize nicks by using your free hand to pull the skin taut. Be patient with each area of skin and keep the blade clog-free by rinsing after every other swipe.

④ **Moisturize afterward.** Shaving removes a very thin top layer of skin, dehydrating you, so apply moisturizing lotion soon after a shave so you'll stay smooth and soft.

⑤ **Sometimes, even well-shaven skin suffers.** In such cases, squeeze a few eyedrops formulated for redness removal directly on your burning bumps. This cheap and effective solution reduces the swelling in a flash!

There are moving dots in
my scalp or pubic hair.

## WHAT'S GOING ON?

Got an itch that can't be scratched? If so, you're one of millions of young adults who find themselves scratching up a storm, unaware that bloodsucking lice have made a home in their hair!

Lice are flat, wingless, bloodsucking parasites that attach themselves and their eggs to body or scalp hair. Head lice and pubic lice are the two main species we deal with, and both look like tiny, moving dots.

Although head lice are most common in young children, people of any age can get them from letting an infected person borrow a hat, comb, brush, towel, clothing, or other personal item. It's even possible to get head lice from sleeping on an infected pillow or couch!

Pubic lice, however, are more of an X-rated issue. They're nearly always spread through sexual contact, and they cause serious itching in the genital area. The slang name for pubic lice is "crabs" because that's exactly what these critters look like.

## HOW DO I DEAL?

Is your skin crawling yet? The first step is to stop freaking out and *see a doctor ASAP.* Although lice aren't life-threatening, the open sores they create can cause infections and leave scars. Head lice can even spread to eyebrows and eyelashes!

Luckily, it's not too hard to get rid of lice. Numerous over-the-counter shampoos and treatments kill lice on your head, and washing your linens and clothes in super-hot water removes any remaining pests.

For pubic lice, a doctor's visit is the best remedy, not only to cure your crabs with prescription medicine but also to be tested for other sexually transmitted infections (STIs) that might not be as obvious.

head lice

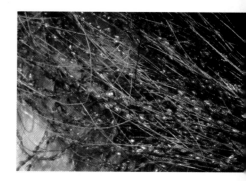

pubic lice

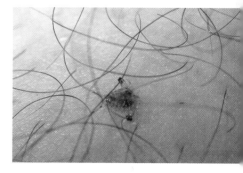

## WHAT IF THEY NOTICE?

If someone spots your pubic problem, good! If they're that close to your private parts, chances are *they* need to be checked out, too.

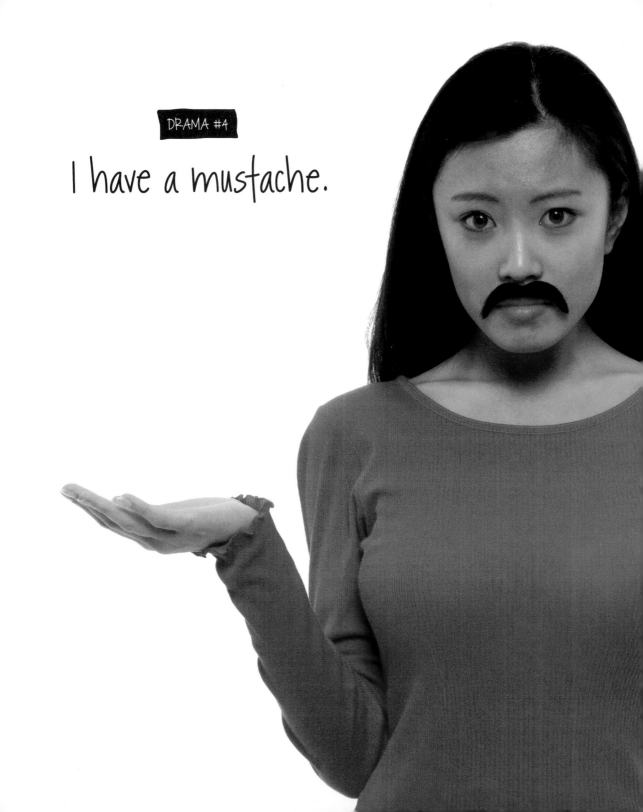

DRAMA #4

# I have a mustache.

## WHAT'S GOING ON?

With over 5 million follicles on the body, there are bound to be a few hairs that pop up in some not-so-expected places. At any time, you might find a new crop of hair on your bottom, a belly button bush, or (what I hate most) a coat of coarse hairs on your chin and upper lip. Many of us even grow nipple nests!

There are two types of body hair: vellus, the peach fuzz that lightly covers most of your entire body; and terminal, the thicker, darker, denser hair that shows up in your armpits, legs, crotch, and other places you might not expect (or want). As your hormones pump while your body continues to change, terminal hair growth can kick into high gear at any time. Only a few places on the body—nails, lips, palms, and the soles of our feet—have no hair follicles. Everywhere else is fair game for future fur!

## HOW DO I DEAL?

Chances are you're going to have hair in some unwanted place at some time in your life. Although some of us freak out over body or facial hair, many women (and their significant others) don't mind it. Body hair removal is a choice that should be made based on your personal preference.

Ask yourself: Is a stray strand or two a big deal? Once started, hair removal is difficult to stop because new growth can often have a more obvious appearance, so be sure that removing your extra fuzz is worth the fuss.

That being said, hair removal is, for many of us, a rite of passage and a way of life. If you decide you're ready to start smoothing out, turn to page 173 for a list of ways to safely remove the hair from different parts of your body, or turn to page 176 for tips on how to choose a safe salon for professional hair removal services.

*fast fact*

*One main function of body hair is to keep our body organs warm and safe. When a person becomes anorexic and stops eating for an extended period of time, the body begins to lack the amount of fat necessary to maintain body temperature. When this happens, in a desperate attempt to protect vital body organs against the cold, a thin layer of body hair called lanugo appears. When enough warming body fat is regained, the lanugo disappears.*

## WHAT IF THEY NOTICE?

Those wispy cheek hairs might seem like a big deal to you in your magnifying mirror, but if you're terrified of the tweezers and wilt at the thought of hot wax, don't worry: They're probably unnoticeable by everyone else. Everyone has extra hair somewhere, but if you're bothered, this book has tons of resources to help you to minimize yours.

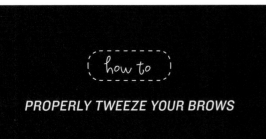

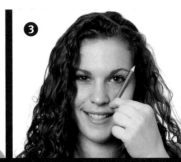

*how to*

### PROPERLY TWEEZE YOUR BROWS

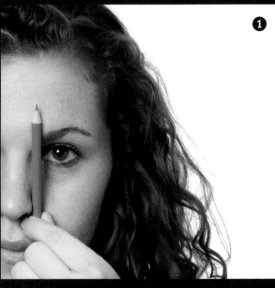

① For full, fabulous brows, look in the mirror and hold a pencil vertically beside the outer edge of your nose. See where it hits? That's your guideline for where your brow should begin. Tweeze any farther in and you'll look overplucked.

② Next, to find where your arch should begin, rotate the pencil over your pupil. If you arch farther up or down your brow, you'll end up looking surprised or depressed.

③ Finally, rotate the pencil until the side stops at the corner of your eye. This is your guideline for where your brow should end.

*Does brow tweezing feel like self-torture? The act of slowly removing hairs one by one with tweezers can be especially painful. To dull the pain, try numbing the area with an ice cube before beginning to tweeze. Also, you can further lessen the pain by creating a smoother hair removal surface. With the hand that is not holding the tweezers, use your fingers to tightly pull your eyebrow skin upward and pluck individual hairs at a slant. With these tips, you'll never tweeze through tears again!*

# HAIR REMOVAL METHODS

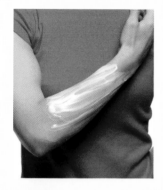

### BLEACHING

Bleaching isn't exactly hair removal, but chemical lightening is a popular method for making body and facial hair less visible without pain. Bleaching is best for arm, chin, and facial hair, but it isn't the best option for dark-skinned individuals because it can make the hair even more visible against their skin. Bleaching has to be done about every four weeks or whenever new hair growth becomes noticeable. The harsh chemicals may provoke an allergic reaction, so those with sensitive skin should steer clear. No matter how desperate you are to match from top to bottom, having harsh chemicals around your private parts is NOT recommended. Bleach "down there" can cause not only skin irritation but also a lot of pain.

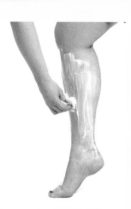

### WAXING

Ever since ancient Egyptians layered their entire bodies with honey and oil and ripped the concoction off with cloth sheets, waxing has been an extremely popular method of hair removal. Like threading and tweezing, waxing pulls the hair out by the root, lengthening the time needed between hair removal sessions. Waxing also removes dead cells from the top layer of the skin, creating a softening effect. It's hard to wax yourself, but it's easy to pick up infections or have a painful experience with this procedure in a salon. Check page 176 for tips on having a positive professional waxing experience.

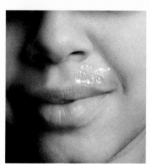

### LOTIONS AND CREAMS

Often called depilatories (the generic term for all types of hair removal), hair removal creams and lotions chemically dissolve hairs at the skin's surface. Most depilatory products call for smearing on the preparation, waiting about ten to fifteen minutes, and then removing the depilatory (and the hair) with a washcloth or paper towel.

Next to trimming, this is the least painful hair removal option, but it's also the messiest. The chemicals make it the smelliest, too. With creams or lotions, you're only removing the surface hair, so the results usually last only about as long as shaving. The chemicals can cause rashes and burns, so before slathering the product on your entire body, patch test a small area of your skin, such as behind your ear, to check for sensitivities.

(Turn to the next page for more methods.)

# HAIR REMOVAL METHODS

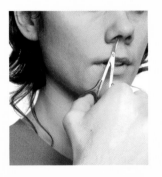

### TRIMMING

Although trimming doesn't completely remove hair, a little bit of landscaping can go a long way. People of all hair types can safely trim at home, and trimming is especially useful for people with sensitive skin and those who are prone to razor bumps. While it's possible to taper any body hair, trimming is especially useful for nipping nose hair (use safety scissors like the ones shown), primping pubic hair, and shaping shaggy eyebrows. Trimming can be done when needed, and it can also be used in combination with some other hair removal methods. For example, trimming long hairs before shaving or waxing makes hair removal much easier (and perhaps unneeded).

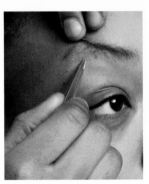

### TWEEZING

Although other methods focus on grooming large patches of hair, tweezing takes a slower, more exact approach by removing entire hairs individually, root and all. Tweezing is best for more sparsely covered areas, such as your chin or toes. Its precision makes it excellent for shaping eyebrows. Tweezing seems painful, perhaps because it goes at a turtle's pace and you can feel each individual pluck. But rushing the process can cause improper tweezing, which leads to scarring and pitting of the skin if you pinch or dig too deeply. You can tweeze hairs whenever, but it's easy to go overboard, leaving you with unnatural, pencil-thin brows that can take forever (if ever!) to grow back. Know when to stop!

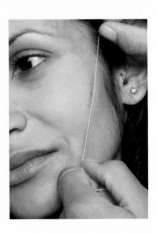

### THREADING

Threading is the Eastern art of removing entire rows of hair at once with two pieces of string strategically wound between the practitioner's fingers. Because it's a speedier version of tweezing that happens to be less expensive, slightly less painful, and much neater than waxing, threading has recently become popular in America for eyebrow shaping and facial hair removal. A popular threading request is for the removal of ALL facial hair, including the forehead, cheeks, ears, and neck. Since the hair is removed from the root, it's possible to stay smooth for up to a month after threading. Because of the constant irritation of the string against the skin, temporary puffiness, soreness, and reddening of the skin are common. People with sensitive skin should start off with a simple eyebrow or chin threading to see how their skin reacts before going for the full face.

## MEDICALLY SUPERVISED HAIR REMOVAL

*If you feel as if your hair removal needs to go beyond the usual techniques, see your doctor for advice on more permanent options, such as prescription medicine to decrease hair growth. Electrolysis and laser treatments permanently remove individual hairs from the root, but to completely smooth an entire area, your doctor will have to treat you quite a few times, making this a VERY expensive option. It's best to consult a doctor before letting anyone zap you, especially if you have darker-toned skin. Thousands of women each year suffer serious burns and scarring from letting unskilled people perform electrolysis or laser hair removal. So, above all, STAY SAFE!*

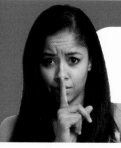

## i confess:
## i had a terrible waxing experience.

I was a sophomore in college and I desperately wanted to get my eyebrows waxed. I was low on cash, so instead of the lovely spa I usually patronized, I decided to save seven dollars by going to a hole-in-the wall that I passed on my way to my internship. The sign outside screamed EYEBROW WAX ONLY $5!!! The moment I walked in, I knew I should have left, but I'd already nodded to the question "Eyebrows?" and was immediately whisked to a tattered chair, where a paper towel was placed over my T-shirt to catch drips. I sat back and got ready. After all, it was only five bucks. How bad could it be? The waxer picked up a Popsicle stick that had probably been sitting in the sloppy, dirty pot of wax all day. Who knows how many people's faces that wax had been spread over? Before I could protest, she spread the wax over my brow, going much higher up than I wanted. The stuff burned terribly, but as I cringed, she just poked the wax until it hardened. Then, R-R-R-RIPP! Up came the wax—and half my eyebrow! To make matters worse, I was BLEEDING! The wax had been too hot, and she had been very rough, making the top layer of my brow skin come off! I ran out crying, skipped my internship, and went to my regular waxer that afternoon. She put a soothing solution on the burn and did her best to even the brows out. It took weeks for the wound to heal and even longer for the hair to grow back, but it was a lesson I'll never forget. I think that it could have been worse. What if I'd gone to that awful place for a bikini wax?

Spas are meant to help you relax and beautify, but ugly infections from unclean salons are on the rise due to untrained technicians. With the increasing popularity of body waxing, manicure, and pedicure services, many unqualified places have popped up. Although their prices might be good, the owners don't keep their businesses up to health code standards, leaving their clients at risk for fungal or bacterial infections.

Before you book an appointment, make sure that the service provider is licensed by your state. If he or she is, you should see a license with a picture and valid expiration date posted somewhere in the store. If you don't, shop around until you find a provider that has the right credentials. That extra five dollars you might spend for safe service is way better than five thousand in medical bills!

*Once you've found a licensed professional, here's how to make sure you're in the right hands:*
*DURING WAXING*

• There should always be a separate cup of wax for each client. Double dipping in a community tub of wax is an easy way to pick up nasty germs and infections.

• There should always be paper covering the waxing table, and it should be fresh and clean.

• If you're having a bikini wax, the technician should always use a new pair of gloves when touching your genitals to minimize the chance of transmitting bacteria and viruses. Even if the practitioner insists that she doesn't need to wear them, you need to stay firm in your request. If she won't comply, leave. Who knows where her hands have been?

• Disposable underwear should be offered to you to put on before waxing your private parts. Human papilloma virus (HPV, page 123) has been found on the underwear of infected individuals.

• The cloth or paper strip the waxer uses to lift the hair should not have another person's hair on it and, if you're having a big patch of hair removed, it should be changed frequently.

• If the waxer grabs scissors or tweezers, ask if the tool has been sterilized or used on another person. If she hesitates even slightly before answering, tell her to keep the instrument away from your skin.

## DURING NAIL SERVICES

• Make sure your technician's license is visible and current.

• Ask to see the tools (including the nail file) before the technician starts working on you. Make sure the implements have been disinfected and sterilized. Otherwise, they could be contaminated, and you'll walk out not only with a French pedicure but also with a toe-threatening staph infection. Many salons will let you bring your own tools or purchase new ones in the shop to ensure sanitary conditions.

• Although legal in some states, getting your cuticles cut or your feet scraped with a razor is not wise. If you allow a technician to perform either procedure, make sure she uses a brand-new blade and sterile cuticle cutters.

• If you're getting a pedicure, make sure the soaking tub has been sprayed with bleach and cleanser. Soaking your feet in a contaminated tub makes you an easy target for invading bacteria or fungi, especially if you recently shaved your legs.

Now that you've nixed the cheap but unsafe places, if a professional manicure or waxing is beyond your budget, check www.nancyredd.com for tips on how to achieve amazing nails and perfect waxing on your own!

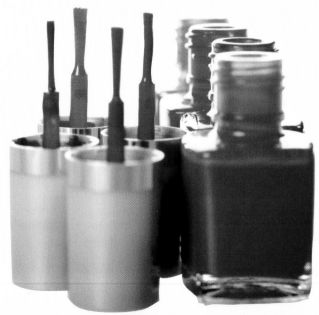

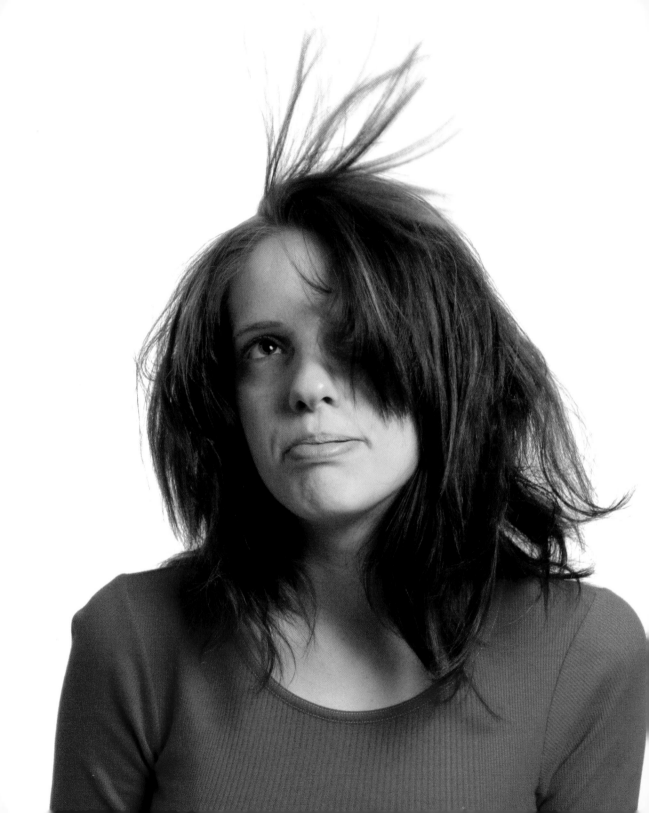

# I fried my hair.

## WHAT'S GOING ON?

Life might sometimes be a little dull, but there are many affordable and temporary ways to make certain that your hair never has to be! Unfortunately, after a disastrous experiment, you might find yourself wishing for the dull 'do days before you accidentally turned your hair into a dry, damaged disaster! Sure, you knew you should have waited six weeks after your last dye job, but you just had to try that new shade of red, leaving your hair completely dead!

Chemical treatments + heated styling tools + hair spray = tons of damage. When used too often or incorrectly, all those products we spend gobs of money on to make us look better can actually make our manes mangy to the point of no return!

It's not just what we do to our hair that can cause damage, but also how we take care of our bodies. Lack of sleep, poor diet, and anxiety can contribute to tragic tresses.

## HOW DO I DEAL?

If you've stressed your strands with a perm or hair dye, start a routine of hair therapy. Immediately lay off the chemicals and lay on the leave-in conditioner, or treat yourself to an at-home, deep-conditioning treatment (see the sidebar on the next page for how).

If you're in the beginning phases of tress therapy, talk to a professional (many hair salons have free consultations) about whether what's hanging from your scalp is salvageable. You might do best to cut off the damaged parts. They're going to break off eventually, anyway.

As hard as it is, try to be patient while waiting for your normal hair to grow. Like anything worthwhile, hair repair takes time. While you're waiting, check your lifestyle habits. Are you super-stressed? Are you getting enough sleep? Staying calm and sleeping at least eight hours a night promote good body health, which in turn helps your hair. Are you eating properly? Certain nutrients and minerals, such as vitamin B12 and sulfur, may stimulate hair growth. You can get these hair helpers from foods such as fish, meat, nuts, eggs, beans, and veggies.

## DEEP CONDITION YOUR HAIR

① Wash your hair with your usual shampoo and drench it in a good conditioner that's right for your hair type, carefully combing through with a wide-toothed comb to ensure even coverage.

② Put on a disposable shower cap.

③ Turn your blow dryer on high and run it back and forth over your cap-covered head until your whole scalp has heated up. Don't wave the blow dryer too close to the cap or it might melt the plastic!

④ Leave the shower cap on for an hour or two before rinsing the conditioner out. Try this treatment once a week and you should soon feel a difference and see improvement.

Once your hair is back to normal, limit your hair experimentation in the future. Although coloring and other chemical treatments are best left to a hair professional you trust, if you can't afford a salon (or simply enjoy doing it yourself), make sure to follow ALL the directions in the package, especially regarding time limits. You have no one to blame except yourself if your hair turns green because you left the color on for thirty minutes instead of three!

## WHAT IF THEY NOTICE?

Tearing your hair out trying to come up with a solution for your limp locks? The best way to avoid calling attention to your problematic pieces (besides wearing a hat) is to gently pull your hair back with a soft elastic band into a neat ponytail. If your hair isn't long enough to pull back, try using bobby pins, headbands, and cute clips to keep it neatly in place until it grows out. While this isn't the most exciting style, it gives your hair a much-needed rest and is always attractive.

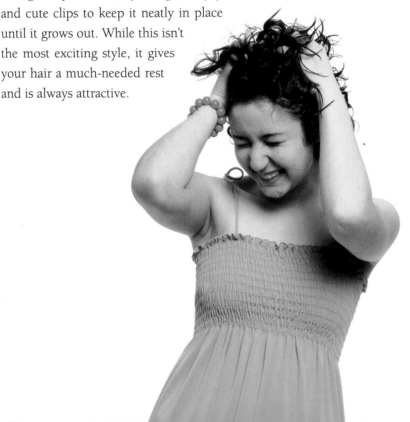

# HAIR LOST & FOUND

Girls never expect to lose their hair, especially in their teens. Unfortunately, it happens more often that you'd think. About 4 million people in America deal with alopecia (al-uh-PEE-shee-uh) areata, the temporary or permanent loss of patches of head hair.

It's normal to shed about a hundred hairs daily, but if you notice small, round, bald scalp spots, or if it seems that more strands than usual are saying sayonara, *see your doctor.* Besides alopecia, there are other conditions that speed up hair loss, such as stress, dieting, illness, and taking certain medications.

Blessed with a thick, healthy head of hair? Consider donating a few of your locks to those who aren't as lucky!

## DONATING YOUR HAIR TO CHARITY

Imagine going bald at the age of thirteen. Unfortunately, because of cancer and other medical reasons, thousands of kids and teens do each year. If you have at least ten inches of hair and are thinking about getting a new 'do, why not donate the leftovers to charity?

Locks of Love is an organization providing hairpieces to youth who have lost their hair. Because it's more socially problematic for young women to be bald, most of the recipients are women.

Interested? Your hair must be in a clean, dry ponytail when snipped, and at least ten inches in length. Also, the more, the better, so get your friends involved! It takes six to ten ten-inch ponytails to make a single wig. For more information and a donation form, check out www.locksoflove.org.

This donor's ponytail helps young women go from this . . .                    to this!

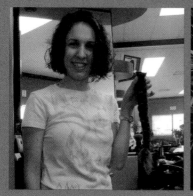
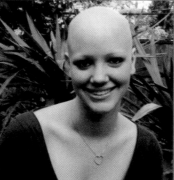
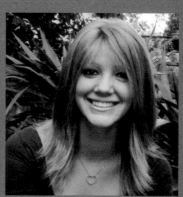

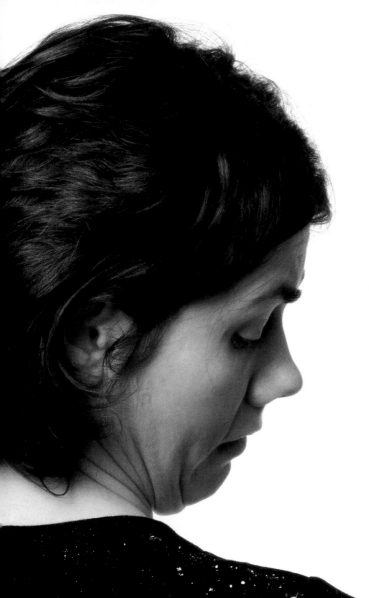

# When I scratch my head, white flakes fall on my clothes.

## WHAT'S GOING ON?

If it's the middle of spring but your shoulders are snowed in, you're probably one of over 50 million folks who get dandruff.

Head confetti tends to come and go in spurts, depending on outside factors. Your scalp skin sheds itself about once a month, but sometimes this process of flaking skin speeds up. Dandruff is an overabundance of dead cells that clump with skin oils, turning into noticeable flakes that take on many different forms. Dandruff can be dusty, shiny, wet, or scaly. Because cold air tends to dry the skin, dandruff is more common in the winter. Stress can also be a major factor in the amount of dandruff you produce: The more you worry, the more you flake!

## HOW DO I DEAL?

Whatever the cause, dandruff is embarrassing and the resulting clumps of oil and dead cells can make your scalp smell nasty, too. Luckily, it's not harmful to your health or contagious, so don't worry about catching it from your brother's baseball cap (though I still wouldn't put it on—ew!).

Sometimes what we mistake for dandruff is residue from hair gels, sprays, or other products. Scalp flakes can even be leftover shampoo or conditioner that wasn't rinsed out properly. If you think product buildup might be the culprit, keeping a clean head of hair, brushing and combing it often, and oiling your scalp, if necessary, can help fend off flakes. Also, there are specific shampoos that can help rinse away leftover hair product flakes.

If it's definitely the real dandruff deal, try an over-the-counter medicated shampoo from the drugstore and minimize the number of hair products you use. If after a few weeks you continue to find crumbles in your comb, *see a doctor*. He or she can give you a prescription shampoo and can check to make sure you don't have a more severe scalp problem, such as psoriasis or seborrheic (**seb-uh-REE-ik**) dermatitis.

## WHAT IF THEY NOTICE?

If you're dealing with dandruff, set aside your black shirts and jackets for the moment, since they make the flakes more noticeable. Wear white and lighter-colored tops until you can get the condition under control.

Frequently check your head for visible pieces that are stuck in your hair. Brush fallen flakes off your shoulders and back often. Also, don't stop washing your hair! It's easy to think that shampooing might be drying out your scalp, but flakes can pile up on a dirty scalp, making the problem worse (and smellier).

If someone spies your scalp and says something rude, blame your dandruff on your hair spray. After all, that might be true!

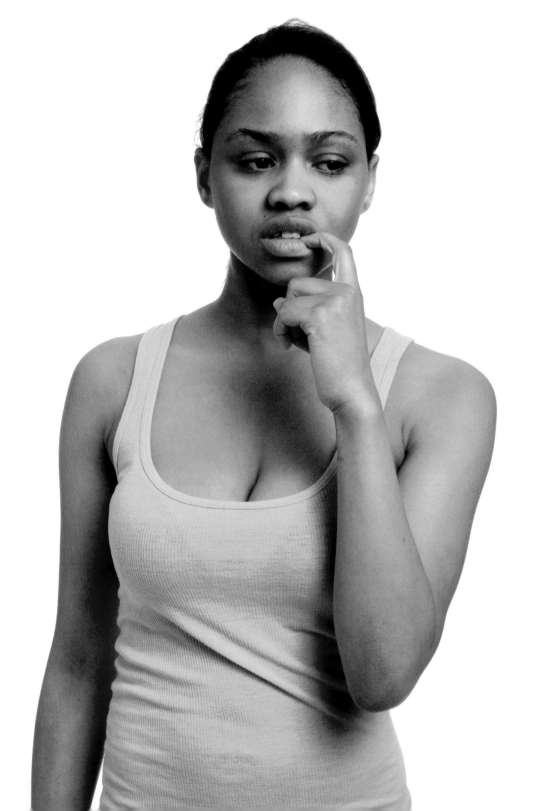

# I chew or pull on my hair or nails all the time.

## WHAT'S GOING ON?

Find yourself tearing your hair out in an effort to stop biting your nails? Everyone has habits adopted as a way of dealing with life. Lots of people fidget, many talk too quickly or loudly, others eat (or don't eat), while some of us take out our frustrations on our hair and nails.

Although chewing, plucking, and tugging might deliver temporary stress relief, constant pulling and nibbling can cause permanent damage. The friction between your hands, mouth, and teeth causes splintered nails, ragged cuticles, or fractured hair shafts. In both your hair and nails, this weakening can cause splitting, breakage, pain, bleeding, infection, and even baldness or nail loss! Unfortunately, the damage is long-lasting; long after you stop, your hair and nails are still a mess.

*fast fact*

*Did you know that nail polish has been around for more than five thousand years? In fact, the color of nails signified social class in ancient China. Only queens were allowed to wear dark polish, and if an ordinary woman was caught in anything other than pale tones, she could be sentenced to death!*

Starting to recognize your hands or hair in this text? Find yourself reaching for a nail or strand to bite on? You're not alone! Lots of us twist and twirl our hair occasionally, half of all adolescents chew their nails, and between 25 and 33 percent of college kids admit to biting.

Sometimes, however, these habits are more than a nervous tic. Extreme nail-biting, medically known as onychophagia **(on-ih-koh-FAY-juh)**, can be a sign of other issues, such as obsessive-compulsive disorder (OCD). *See your doctor* if you're concerned about your habits.

Think you're an extreme hair puller? Between 1 and 2 percent of Americans suffer from a psychological disorder medically known as trichotillomania **(trik-uh-til-uh-MAY-nee-uh)**. People with trichotillomania may find themselves doing more than twisting, chewing, and pulling on their scalp hair. To release tension, sufferers may be addicted to plucking their eyebrows, eyelashes, leg, arm, and even pubic hair, not stopping regardless of the pain, leading to bald spots, bleeding fingers, and scarring.

## HOW DO I DEAL?

Finding yourself with a mouth or handful of hair more often than you'd like? Want to nip the nibbling in the bud? If you're twisting from tension or biting in boredom, try to pinpoint what exactly triggers the habit. Once you've figured it out, consider substituting a new, less problematic habit, such as squeezing a stress ball, chewing sugarless gum, or keeping your hands busy with something else when that craving comes.

If substitution or willpower won't work, try the "out-of-sight, out-of-mouth" approach by wearing your hair in a ponytail (away from your hands and mouth). Or make the habit less appealing by using a nasty-tasting shampoo or by dipping your fingers in black pepper, vinegar, or other bitter-tasting creams or solutions. Just make sure they're safe to ingest in case you still can't resist! Your drugstore should have some nasty-tasting nontoxic formulas made for nail-biters.

*fast fact*

*Fingernails grow up to twice as fast as toenails, especially in the winter.*

Another way to solve the problem is to give yourself a great hairstyle or manicure. This not only helps to repair the damage, but the perfect 'do or pretty polish might also discourage chewing!

If you think you're suffering from severe nail-biting or trichotillomania, *see your doctor* or school counselor to get something (besides hair) off your chest! Your doctor can determine how much, if any, damage has already been done to your skin, hair, or nails and can prescribe medication or refer you to a specialist if additional help is needed.

**F.Y.I.**

# NAIL COLOR AND HEALTH

Your eyes may be mirrors into your soul, but your nails are mirrors into your health! The color of your nail bed can help doctors diagnose certain serious illnesses. *See your doctor* to determine if these conditions are the culprit of your nail color.

| COLOR | ILLNESS |
|---|---|
| Yellowing with a bluish base | Diabetes |
| Paler than normal | Anemia |
| Half white, half pink | Kidney problems |
| White | Liver problems |

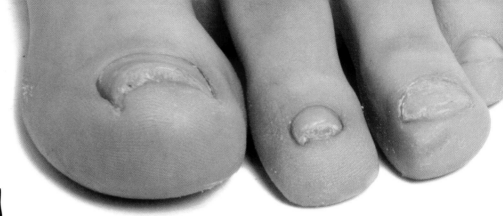

# I have yucky stuff underneath my nails.

## WHAT'S GOING ON?

Do you feel as if you're in a (toe) jam when it comes to the condition of your feet? Though all of us get a bit of dirt under our nails from time to time, actual fungus of the nail, known as onychomycosis **(ahn-ee-koh-my-KOH-sis)**, is a common occurrence on both your fingers and toes, though it's ten times more likely to appear on your tootsies. Symptoms include a nasty stench and crumbly, funny-colored bits attached to your skin and nails. Lost your appetite yet?

Any nail in a moist, dark environment is fair game. Don't think those sweaty socks are the only popular breeding ground! Going swimming with acrylic fingernails and not drying your hands well are also fungus-friendly habits. Sometimes you don't even have to leave the nail salon to get infected — an unclean salon can be an open market for onychomycosis on your fingers or toes (see page 176 for tips on avoiding an unsafe situation).

Besides the visible, stinky problems, you may also experience itching and in some cases pain. Shoes that rub your toenails may become uncomfortable to wear.

## HOW DO I DEAL?

The first step is to air out the situation. If you've been hiding the fungus under fake nails, nail polish, or in closed-toe shoes, remove them immediately. Giving your skin room to breathe and keeping your nails clean and dry are the only way you'll ever heal.

While there are over-the-counter treatments available, it's hard to get rid of a fungal infection on your own. *See your doctor* to find out how advanced your case is. A physician can prescribe medication that will help solve the problem faster.

DRAMA #9

My teeth aren't white.

# WHAT'S GOING ON?

The glamorous grins you see in magazines and on TV can understandably make your own smiles seem sallow, but those sparkling celebrity smiles are usually the result of false teeth, porcelain veneers, and some pretty powerful bleach.

Naturally occurring perfect, pearly whites are actually more pearly than white. That's because the exposed parts of our teeth have two important parts: the outer enamel, which is translucent; and the layer beneath it, which is called dentin. Dentin is light yellow. Light that passes through the enamel is reflected by the dentin, giving teeth a pearly color.

Dark pigments from coffee, tea, colas, and staining foods like blueberries can be deposited on our translucent outer tooth enamel. Also, smoking cigarettes contributes heavily to tooth staining (yet another reason not to smoke!), making teeth look brown or yellow.

*fast fact*

*Are veneers really false teeth? Kinda! A veneer is a thin shell (usually of porcelain) that is glued to the front side of an individual tooth that has been sanded down to make room. Some people get them to cover up spaces, chips, and cracks, while others choose them over braces. Today, some people (and many celebrities) get veneers simply because it's impossible to get real teeth a blinding shade of white. People will do anything for beauty!*

## HOW DO I DEAL?

The naturally creamy coloration of teeth was hardly questioned until veneers (false fronts installed on top of natural teeth) and tooth-whitening substances (found in everything from chewing gum to toothpaste to specialized whitening strips) became so popular.

Before branching out to beaming teeth, figure out if your teeth *really* need to be whitened. Some people might look worse with marshmallow-white teeth! Experts say your teeth shouldn't be whiter than the whites of your eyes. If they are, you'll look tired and sick.

Notice dark places on your teeth? Before whitening, see your dentist to make sure that the discoloration is staining and not the beginning stages of a cavity or other tooth damage. If the dentist gives you the go-ahead, try an over-the-counter bleaching kit or oral hygiene product with whitener in it before plunking down the cash for a professional job. Often you can get the results you want after just a few applications. As you become more satisfied with your sparkling smile, try not to become too obsessed. Excessive whitening can weaken your enamel, in turn darkening your teeth!

Try preventing future darkening by drinking darker liquids out of a straw to minimize contact with your teeth, but don't try that with hot coffee! To make the most of what you have, if you wear lipstick, choose colors with bluish undertones instead of yellows. A purple-pink lipstick color will make your teeth appear whiter and brighter than a golden neutral shade.

And, if you're smoking, STOP! If you don't quit soon, dirty-looking teeth will be the least of your problems. See page 193 for reasons why.

If you're under the age of fourteen, *do not* whiten your teeth. Your teeth are still pushing out of your gums and haven't yet reached their full length. As tempting as tooth whitening may be, the last thing you need is a permanently two-toned tooth! Stick to whitening toothpastes, which are safe for almost everyone to use.

**F.Y.I.**

# BRACES

Brace yourself: Dentists estimate that 75 percent of us could benefit from braces, and that 4.5 million Americans are currently wearing them. Are you a "Brace Face"? If so, your parents' experiences with braces was probably a lot different from yours. Only a few years ago, clunky, metal mouth ornaments brought about tons of teasing for the unfortunate wearer. New strides in braces technology, ranging from invisible braces to colored bands you can coordinate with your clothes, as well as the general popularity of tooth correction, has made braces a popular and common part of growing up. Many kids are now teased if they DON'T wear braces! That's not fair either, for braces can be expensive—up to $5,000 a jaw!

If you're part of the braces community, there are a few extra steps you'll need to take to keep your breath fresh and your teeth clean and free of cavities. Always brush immediately after eating. Floss and gargle frequently. Since you can't chew gum to remove particles and keep your saliva flowing, keep with you at all times a small mirror, toothpicks, and special flossing sticks formulated to get between teeth and braces easily. Don't worry, all this extra care will be worth the effort once the braces come off!

Have your braces already come off? If so, wear your retainer! Otherwise, your teeth will shift back to their original, crooked positions, and all those years of repair will go down the drain in just a short while.

# My breath is HARSH!

## WHAT'S GOING ON?

Is my outfit perfect? Check. How's my hair? Great. Do my pits smell? Nope. How's my breath? OH NO! Sometimes, instead of our beauty leaving people breathless, our mouth odor, medically known as halitosis **(hal-i-TOH-sis)**, might turn others off.

As we all know, certain strong-smelling foods (such as garlic or coffee) can cause bad breath that lasts for hours. Still, yesterday's fried onions might not be the culprit of today's oral odors. Instead, the problem might be a bit of this morning's breakfast stuck behind your molars! Food often gets stuck between teeth, and even if we can't feel it, others can smell it as it decomposes in our mouths. ICK! Untreated cavities, gum disease, smoking cigarettes, and alcohol consumption are also common causes of terrible breath.

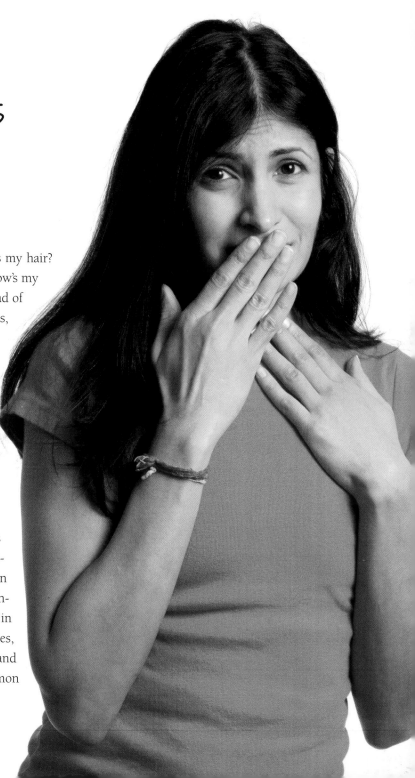

## HOW DO I DEAL?

Everyone knows not to eat a garlic bagel right before a big date, but there are lots of other ways you can give bad breath the heave-ho. A dry mouth is an excellent place for bacteria to fester, producing a funk. In fact, the main cause of "morning breath" is the fact that at night, your spit production slows down, causing your mouth to dry out. Drinking plenty of water and chewing sugarless gum will keep your saliva flowing and help remove food particles from your mouth.

Brushing (with toothpaste, of course) at least twice a day will solve much of your mouth odor. When you're brushing your teeth, don't forget to brush your tongue. Tongues trap odor-causing food particles and bacteria.

Gargling with mouthwash and flossing daily are also good ways to help prevent bad breath. They get rid of bacteria and stuck food particles. Snacking on crunchy raw veggies, such as carrots and celery, is also an excellent way to clean your teeth—and get your vitamins!

Keep emergency breath fresheners in your backpack or purse, including sugarless gum, a travel-size toothbrush, floss, or even a small bottle of mouthwash. The next time your lunchtime salad is unexpectedly tossed with onions, you'll be prepared!

For long-term mouth health, keep in touch with your dentist. A cleaning twice a year will help prevent gum disease, plaque, and tartar buildup, all of which can muck up your mouth. If you still can't get rid of your bad breath and you're certain it's not related to your food or hygiene, *see your doctor* about potential health complications that have chronic halitosis as a side effect, such as a sinus or lung infection, or even diabetes. And, of course, DON'T SMOKE! A smoker's breath smells no matter what.

## WHAT IF THEY NOTICE?

Sometimes our bad breath will be offensive to others, unbeknownst to us. If someone alerts you about your stinky smile, don't get mad at the messenger. Express appreciation for the warning, blame the odor on your breakfast, and ask around for a mint or some gum.

If no breath fresheners are available, try rinsing your mouth with water to loosen food particles. In a pinch, you might also use your finger—clean, of course—as a temporary toothbrush!

# SMOKING
# KILLS

Although everyone knows the negative effects smoking has not only on our skin, teeth, and breath, but also on our lives, about one in five teens are currently regular smokers. According to the American Cancer Society, over 3,000 teenagers start this expensive, dangerous habit each day. Twenty of these smokers will be murdered in their lifetime, thirty will die in car accidents, but more than 750 will die from SMOKING!

*In case you've forgotten, here is a list of the awful effects of smoking:*

- causes DEATH
- causes cancer, heart disease, emphysema, and other medical problems
- slows your body's ability to heal
- causes acne, wrinkles, and leathery skin
- increases risk for going blind
- dulls your taste buds
- causes chronic bad breath
- makes your entire body and all your clothes reek
- leaves you short of breath

Did you notice that smoking KILLS you? Or that it makes your entire body and breath STINK? Seriously, who wants to kiss an ashtray?

If you need help quitting, visit www.nancyredd.com for tips and support or call the American Cancer Society's toll-free Quitline at 1-877-YES-QUIT or visit www.cancer.org.

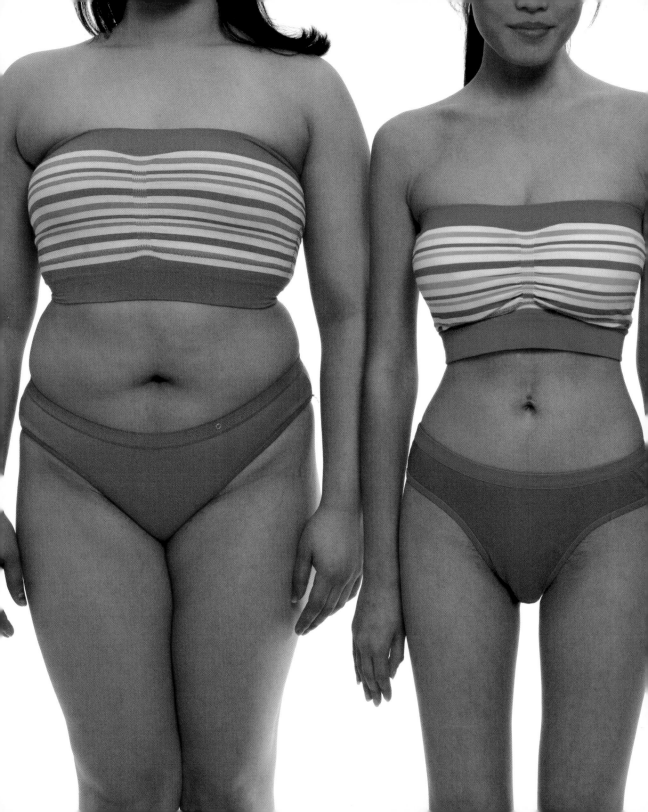

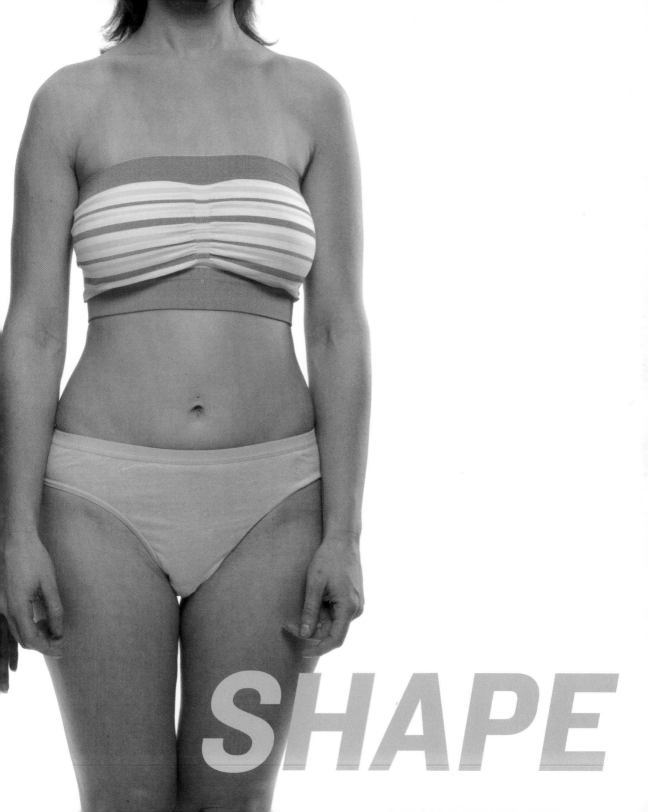

SHAPE

Hovering around one hundred and fifty pounds, wearing a size twelve, and standing five feet, four inches tall, as a senior in high school I was what traditional medical charts consider overweight . . . but I never knew it! Being southern and black meant that a couple of extra inches to pinch were nothing to be ashamed of. At the very worst of times, when I struggled to find a pair of jeans that stretched over my ample behind, I thought of myself as "thickly built," but mostly I just thought of myself as hot stuff.

That same butt that couldn't get into blue jeans could definitely shake it on the dance floor, and my boyfriend never told me I was fat, nor did any of the people in my high school who voted me school president. I was so confident that I even entered a local beauty pageant and won the title, along with sponsorship to the state program! That, however, was where the fairy tale began to unravel.

On the first day of the state competition, I looked around and what I saw shocked me. The vast majority of the other girls were five feet seven inches tall and above, and ALL of them were at least twenty pounds lighter than I was. Soon we were all squished together on the floor in white slips and heels, wondering what would happen next. "Alrightie, girls," the pageant director squealed, "let's see those beautiful dresses, shall we?" We all had to wear the exact same dress, but we got to choose the color. Used to standing out in a good way, I chose watermelon—a loud pink that resembled the color of Pepto-Bismol. After we got dressed, the director asked each of us for our dress size, making sure everything was in order for the other costuming. The other girls chimed in with their sizes in perky, proud voices, "Four!" "Two!" "Six, or four, depending on the bust (giggle)!" When my name was called, I whispered, "Size twelve," hoping no one would hear me, praying that no one would laugh, extremely aware of the fact that I was the only double-digit size in the entire pageant. I dreaded having to wear my humongous, tonsil-colored dress among the sea of tiny burgundies, petite greens, and skinny blues.

At the dinner buffet line, while I filled my plate with "comfort food," I noticed all the other girls took only lettuce. During practices, while everyone else wore sports bras and tiny shorts, I wore a baggy T-shirt and sweats. As the week progressed, I felt weirder and wider and uglier and larger. In my hometown, I may have been a normal seventeen-year-old girl, but here, I was FAT, and fat people

*While weight will come and go, your body shape will stay more or less the same after your body is done growing. A pancake butt will probably stay flat no matter how much weight you gain, and those broad shoulders aren't budging no matter what diet you pursue.*

*You really CAN thank (or blame) your parents for your body shape. A person's frame and body makeup are genetic. Even in the womb, the general shape that each body part will develop in adult life is already predetermined.*

*Peeved when you find that even a size ten won't fit when you're usually a perfect eight? Don't worry! It happens to us all. Each clothing designer chooses his or her own standard for sizing. Some designers size their clothing smaller, while others leave room to spare.*

were not pageant queens. A pageant winner does not go back for a second helping at dinner. I was ashamed and embarrassed for being so different.

It was then that I, Nancy Redd, school president, public speaking champion, and cheerleading captain, began to COMPLETELY hate my EN-TIRE BODY. I had just been accepted into an Ivy League college, and I had a wonderful life back home, but I still felt like a total loser. After the pageant was over, I poured all the energy that had gone into college applications and schoolwork into low-fat cooking and exercising to the point of exhaustion. I lost four dress sizes before I went to college! Much to my disappointment, thanks to stress, laziness, and college cafeteria food, I gained all the weight back by my junior year.

I vowed not to have another senior year like my high school one, so the roller coaster continued as I dusted off my George Foreman grill, pulled out my yoga mat, and painstakingly turned my entire summer into a one-track weight-loss plan. I lost the weight all over again—and then some—going on to win the swimsuit competition at the Miss America Pageant. Still, I constantly felt (and STILL feel!) incredibly uncomfortable with my body, always obsessing over my "problem areas" that are invisible to everyone but me.

It makes me angry to think of how I could once look in the mirror and not see fleshy arms or jiggly thighs. Sadly, with the weight, I lost a special innocence with which I loved myself unconditionally. Even today, I often feel an empty pang in my stomach that isn't from lack of food; it stems from a different kind of hunger: I wonder if size six Nancy is as happy as size twelve Nancy was . . . at half my size, do I love myself half as much?

This chapter was the hardest one for me to write, which probably makes it the most important chapter of all. Facing your own body issues is truly tough—I should know. After years of hard work, I've finally become more comfortable with who I am and how my body is supposed to look. It is extremely liberating! Shape dramas come from the most shameful spaces in our minds and relate to our innermost feelings about these complicated bodies we simultaneously love, hate, and abuse. It's time to put an end to the cycle of self-hate and shame. Now is the time to be open, honest, and proactive about dealing with our shape dramas!

*Think twice before "super-sizing" your burger combo! A recent study found that over a lifetime, each sixty-seven cent fast food meal upgrade ends up costing a woman over THREE DOLLARS due to medical and other complications. So you might think you're saving money by upgrading from medium to large for mere pennies, but the subsequent weight gain and health problems will end up costing you way more.*

*Women are built to have more body fat than men, and we store almost 10 billion more fat cells in our bodies. That isn't a fluke. It's a necessity! We need extra fat cells to menstruate and to reproduce healthily. In fact, if a woman's body fat dips below 17 percent, often her period will stop!*

**DRAMA #1**

I feel fat.

## WHAT'S GOING ON?

Feeling fat is SUCH a head trip. Only 16 percent of teenage girls are overweight, but emotionally, many of us FEEL fat, regardless of whether we truly are. Actually, 14 percent of girls who are perfectly healthy weights for their heights still think of themselves as overweight!

We've all felt fat. The reason might be that extra donut you've been munching on each afternoon for the past month, a little water retention a few days before your period, or a growth spurt that sent your favorite jeans to the charity pile. Or, there might be no reason at all!

Even if we don't really think we're fat, the phrase still spills out like a guilty confession: "OMG, I'm sooo fat!" Feeling "fat" is used as a way to bond with others or even to fish for compliments. "Me too! I'm like mega-fat." "Girl, no you aren't! You look great." "No I don't! I totally need to lose some of this chub." "What chub?" "THIS CHUB!" And the cycle goes on and on until someone changes the subject. What we don't always realize, however, is that the more we torture ourselves with that three-letter word, the more of a problem it becomes.

Society's not helping us by selling clothing draped on size triple-zero models whose pictures have still been airbrushed! How are we supposed to know that someone digitally removed her ribcage and pantyline on a computer, making the outfit appear to drape perfectly on her?

## HOW DO I DEAL?

The number one rule is to remember that feeling fat is not the same as being overweight. Wonder if you could stand to lose a few pounds? Check out the BMI chart on the next page to find out a healthy weight range for you.

# BODY MASS INDEX

The Body Mass Index (BMI) was created in the mid-nineteenth century to give doctors a standard way to gauge a person's body fat using his or her height and weight. Since a six-foot-one girl should weigh more than one who's five foot two, finding your BMI is the best way to figure out the healthiest weight for you.

To determine your BMI, on the chart below move your finger down the column on the left until you find your height in inches. Stop. Now move your finger across that row to the right to find your weight in pounds. Stop again. Now move your finger UP the column until you hit the blue bar. The white number on the blue bar shows your BMI.

If your BMI is less than 19, you are underweight. If it is between 19 and 25, you are at a healthy weight. If it is between 25 and 30, you are overweight. And if your BMI is 30 or over, you are considered obese. Worried about your BMI? *See your doctor.*

## BODY MASS INDEX TABLE

| BMI | 19 | 20 | 21 | 22 | 23 | 24 | 25 | 26 | 27 | 28 | 29 | 30 | 31 | 32 | 33 | 34 | 35 | 36 | 37 | 38 | 39 |
|---|---|---|---|---|---|---|---|---|---|---|---|---|---|---|---|---|---|---|---|---|---|
| Height (inches) | | | | | | | | | | Body Weight (pounds) | | | | | | | | | | | |
| 58 | 91 | 96 | 100 | 105 | 110 | 115 | 119 | 124 | 129 | 134 | 138 | 143 | 148 | 153 | 158 | 162 | 167 | 172 | 177 | 181 | 186 |
| 59 | 94 | 99 | 104 | 109 | 114 | 119 | 124 | 128 | 133 | 138 | 143 | 148 | 153 | 158 | 163 | 168 | 173 | 178 | 183 | 188 | 196 |
| 60 | 97 | 102 | 107 | 112 | 118 | 123 | 128 | 133 | 138 | 143 | 148 | 153 | 158 | 163 | 168 | 174 | 179 | 184 | 189 | 194 | 199 |
| 61 | 100 | 106 | 111 | 116 | 122 | 127 | 132 | 137 | 143 | 148 | 153 | 158 | 164 | 169 | 174 | 180 | 185 | 190 | 195 | 201 | 206 |
| 62 | 104 | 109 | 115 | 120 | 126 | 131 | 136 | 142 | 147 | 153 | 158 | 164 | 169 | 175 | 180 | 186 | 191 | 196 | 202 | 207 | 213 |
| 63 | 107 | 113 | 118 | 124 | 130 | 135 | 141 | 146 | 152 | 158 | 163 | 169 | 175 | 180 | 186 | 191 | 197 | 203 | 208 | 214 | 220 |
| 64 | 110 | 116 | 122 | 128 | 134 | 140 | 145 | 151 | 157 | 163 | 169 | 174 | 180 | 186 | 192 | 197 | 204 | 209 | 215 | 221 | 227 |
| 65 | 114 | 120 | 126 | 132 | 138 | 144 | 150 | 156 | 162 | 168 | 174 | 180 | 186 | 192 | 198 | 204 | 210 | 216 | 222 | 228 | 234 |
| 66 | 118 | 124 | 130 | 136 | 142 | 148 | 155 | 161 | 167 | 173 | 179 | 186 | 192 | 198 | 204 | 210 | 216 | 223 | 229 | 235 | 241 |
| 67 | 121 | 127 | 134 | 140 | 146 | 153 | 159 | 166 | 172 | 178 | 185 | 191 | 198 | 204 | 211 | 217 | 223 | 230 | 236 | 242 | 249 |
| 68 | 125 | 131 | 138 | 144 | 151 | 158 | 164 | 171 | 177 | 184 | 190 | 197 | 203 | 210 | 216 | 223 | 230 | 236 | 243 | 249 | 256 |
| 69 | 128 | 135 | 142 | 149 | 155 | 162 | 169 | 176 | 182 | 189 | 196 | 203 | 209 | 216 | 223 | 230 | 236 | 243 | 250 | 257 | 263 |
| 70 | 132 | 139 | 146 | 153 | 160 | 167 | 174 | 181 | 188 | 195 | 202 | 209 | 216 | 222 | 229 | 236 | 243 | 250 | 257 | 264 | 271 |
| 71 | 136 | 143 | 150 | 157 | 165 | 172 | 179 | 186 | 193 | 200 | 208 | 215 | 222 | 229 | 236 | 243 | 250 | 257 | 265 | 272 | 279 |
| 72 | 140 | 147 | 154 | 162 | 169 | 177 | 184 | 191 | 199 | 206 | 213 | 221 | 228 | 235 | 242 | 250 | 258 | 265 | 272 | 279 | 287 |

| *HEALTHY WEIGHT* | *OVERWEIGHT* | *OBESE* |
|---|---|---|

Notice there's no one weight that's right for your height. That's because everyone's body has different amounts of muscle and fat. There is no ONE right number, but there is a range of weights that are healthy for your frame. Everyone's weight fluctuates, but weight change is *not* the same as getting fat.

Next, check your pants! If you're upset because yesterday you had to buy a size eight instead of your usual size six jeans, you may have put on a few pounds since the last time you went shopping (or the pants just might be a different brand, see page 197 for an explanation), but that doesn't make you fat. If you have a muffin top in a pair of jeans that fit you two years ago, you're not fat; you just need to size up. Your body is not supposed to stay the same size forever!

Finally, check your 'tude! Even if you're jokingly moaning about your body being too big, a tiny part of you believes it's true. Perhaps you feel more comfortable about yourself when you're at the lower end of the normal range, and that's understandable, but that's no reason to tear yourself down. Remember, the average American woman weighs 163 pounds and is five feet four inches tall!

If the BMI table shows that you're in a normal range, start looking at your body in a positive light and be thankful for the healthy body that you have! By being negative, you risk psyching yourself out about what you REALLY look like. However, if your BMI confirms that you might have some weight to lose, move on to the next drama for help!

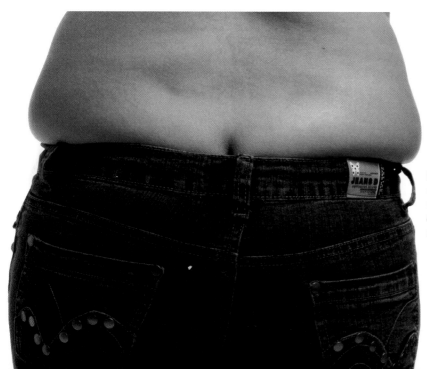

fast fact

*What's a "muffin top"? It's when too-tight jeans cut into the wearer's waist, causing excess fat to spill out over the top, similar to how the top of a muffin puffs over its paper container. You can completely avoid muffin top by wearing pants that are the right size for you, not the size you wish you were.*

# WHAT IS BODY IMAGE?

Put simply, it's the way we think about our physical appearance. A person with a "great" body image feels comfortable and confident with her body most of the time, while a person with a "bad" body image thinks of herself as ugly or unattractive and feels insecure about her body most of the time.

Body image is complicated because it can simultaneously have nothing and everything to do with your actual physical appearance. Even if you're voted "Most Beautiful" by your classmates, you may still feel like the grossest person on the planet.

Say Jane is a smart, healthy, fit, red-haired girl who grows up in an environment where big feet are considered beautiful, but she wears only a size-five shoe. She is likely to feel inadequate about her tiny feet, affecting her body image. Jane is ridiculously jealous of Judy, her pen pal who lives across the world and wears a size-eleven shoe. However, Judy couldn't care less about her feet. In her country, redheads reign, and as a brunette she feels pretty plain looking, so her body image suffers as well.

Body image = a mixture of what society TELLS us we should look like + what we WANT to look like + whether we LIKE what we look like + what we THINK others THINK we look like . . . and the list goes on and on. If Jane and Judy switched places, both might feel more comfortable with themselves at first. But as cultural norms and perceptions of beauty change (and they always do), they may find themselves feeling inadequate about some OTHER part of their body, sending that great new pride back down again.

It's easy to stress out about how others might judge you, and feeling great about your body 100 percent of the time is impossible—*everyone* has bad body days. Still, you have to realize that it is up to YOU, and not your friends or the media, to feel good about yourself and your body. Shifting your mind-set about what is and isn't beautiful, and about how a healthy body is supposed to look, will have a tremendous impact on the rest of your life. A positive, confident attitude about your own uniquely beautiful shape will make you feel much happier no matter what's going on around you, and it can completely change others' perceptions about you. So, give it a shot!

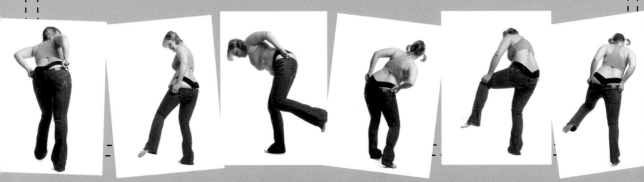

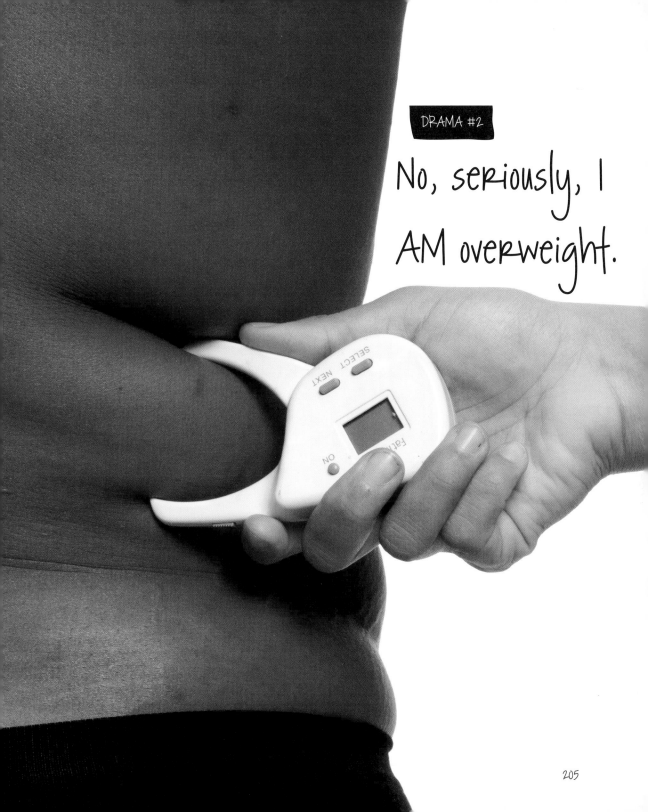

DRAMA #2

No, seriously, I AM overweight.

## WHAT'S GOING ON?

So, does your BMI show that you could stand to lose some weight? If so, you have lots of company! Although the diet industry is booming, Americans are becoming heavier at younger ages each year, and more than 60 percent of adult Americans are overweight.

You might be one of the heavier people among your peers, making you feel different and perhaps embarrassed. On the other hand, you might be as lucky as I was growing up! In many parts of the country, thin is NOT in, and super-curvy bodies are the norm.

No matter what, there can always be too much of a good thing. Carrying around excess weight is not good for your health and overall wellness. Heavy teens can turn into overweight and unhealthy young adults. Extra pounds don't just weigh your body down; they also affect your long-term health. Diabetes, high blood pressure, and shortened life expectancy are just a few of the complications that come from carrying around too many extra pounds. However, how you FEEL is equally as important: Being overweight can leave you sluggish and low on energy, and it can also stress you out. Who needs that?

## HOW DO I DEAL?

Everyone's genetic makeup is different, and we aren't all meant to be thin. Still, eating healthy foods and working out often are very important to our well-being, though sometimes they're easier said than done.

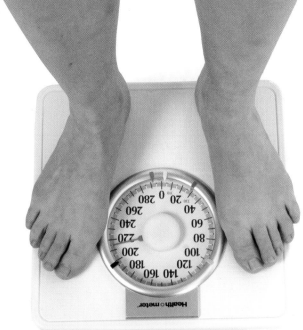

Admittedly, the idea of losing weight and becoming physically fit can be overwhelming. Your weight is more than just a number; it's a part of you! Advice on weight loss isn't what this book is about—there are tons of ways to eat less and exercise more. But what is often forgotten is the importance of making sure your mind is in the right place while you're working on your body. Make sure you're losing the weight for the right reasons—your health and personal satisfaction— not because someone called you "fatty." To lose weight the right way and to stay healthy, you need a more positive motivation than that! By starting a healthy life now, you'll gain confidence—not excess weight! It won't be easy, but it WILL be worth it!

*Ready to get started? Here are some tips:*
**Don't rush in.** Hurrying into the first fad diet you can think of is a *bad* idea. If you start restricting your food too much or try an exercise routine that is too challenging for you, you'll soon crash and burn. You're much more likely to follow through to the end if you slowly start eating better and exercising more often. Try thirty minutes of exercise two days a week to start, then try to increase from there.

**Ask for help.** Haven't a clue how to get in shape? Asking a professional for advice on nipping your weight problem in the bud is an excellent first step. Getting healthy isn't something you should attempt alone, especially if you have a lot to lose. It helps to have someone to talk to about your concerns and to chart your progress along the way. Your parents or guardian, school nurse or counselor, and doctor are all excellent resources to set you on the path to optimal health. They may offer advice, give you a suggested diet and exercise plan, or refer you to a nutritionist for more help. Also, if you know another young woman who could stand to shape up, consider inviting her to join you during workouts. The buddy system is a great way to stay motivated.

**Don't give up.** It didn't take two days for you to gain it all, and it's not going to fall off that quickly, either. Instead of focusing only on the scale and your clothing size, set your sights on maintaining a beautiful, healthy physique. Once you start getting fit, you'll realize that there are many benefits that enhance your entire life, such as extra energy, newfound strength, increased self-confidence, better health, and much more. It takes time, patience, and dedication to get in shape the right way, so celebrate the small stuff: your first five pounds lost, your favorite pants feeling a little looser, a compliment from someone you admire. There are so many things along the way to look forward to!

## WHAT IF THEY NOTICE?

Extra weight is an easy target, making it easy for people to be mean to you just because you have more inches to pinch. Even once you're looking healthier and feeling more confident, people might start ragging on you for that, so be prepared to laugh them off and keep on working! Remember, changing sizes won't change who you are on the inside . . . and it certainly won't change other people's mean tendencies, either! When people take notice positively, use those good feelings to get you through the harder times. And remember, it's how *you* feel at the end of the day that matters most.

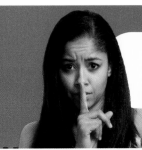

## i confess:
## people can be mean.

When I went back to college my senior year after my summer of getting in shape, I was totally crushed by some of my friends' reactions to my new bod. While most people were supportive and proud of me, surprisingly, there was a lot of negativity. Some people made fun of me to my face, while others talked about me behind my back. Really mean things were said that hurt my feelings. It's no fun when the feedback from all your hard work isn't 100 percent positive, but in life, you're going to have some naysayers—especially when you're working hard to better yourself. Try not to let other people's negativity sway your opinions about yourself and don't start giving up or trying to change yourself in an attempt to please others. Your weight loss is for YOU to become healthier and to feel more confident, not for anyone else. Even if you're perfect (which I think you are anyway), something can always be found to pick on and something mean can always be said, so stay focused on your goal of self-improvement and self-acceptance.

# I want to get fit and eat right, but it's expensive!

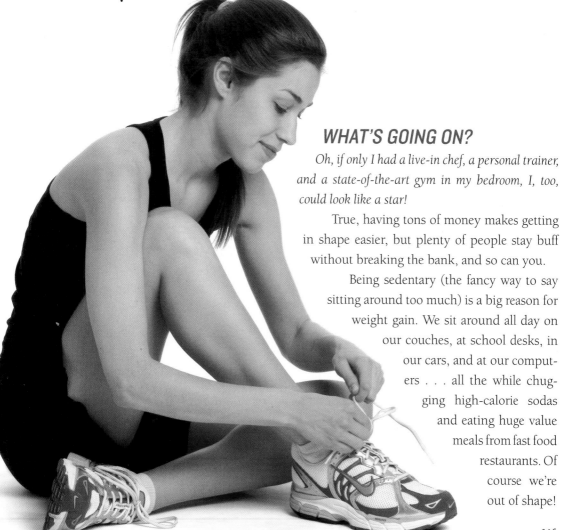

## WHAT'S GOING ON?

*Oh, if only I had a live-in chef, a personal trainer, and a state-of-the-art gym in my bedroom, I, too, could look like a star!*

True, having tons of money makes getting in shape easier, but plenty of people stay buff without breaking the bank, and so can you.

Being sedentary (the fancy way to say sitting around too much) is a big reason for weight gain. We sit around all day on our couches, at school desks, in our cars, and at our computers . . . all the while chugging high-calorie sodas and eating huge value meals from fast food restaurants. Of course we're out of shape!

Weight loss is simply a numbers game. The amount of energy found in food is measured in calories. If you consume more calories than you burn each day, you gain weight. If you burn more calories than you eat each day, you'll slim down. Simple as that! While advertisements make us think that there's no way we can get in shape without expensive supplements and equipment, in reality losing weight and getting fit have nothing to do with money. Remember, many of those stars worked hard on their bodies *before* they made it big enough to hire pricey help.

## HOW DO I DEAL?

It's easy to come up with excuses not to exercise, and being unable to afford a gym membership is a common one. But since calories can be burned any-where, this excuse won't work! There are only two elements of success-ful weight loss: exercise and eating healthily.

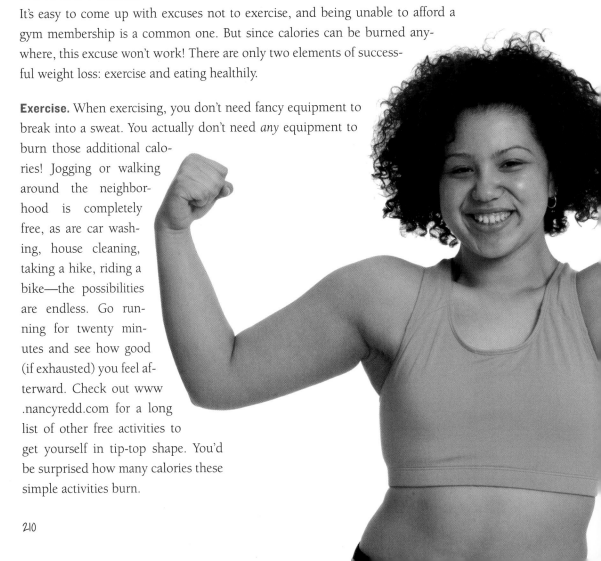

**Exercise.** When exercising, you don't need fancy equipment to break into a sweat. You actually don't need *any* equipment to burn those additional calories! Jogging or walking around the neighborhood is completely free, as are car washing, house cleaning, taking a hike, riding a bike—the possibilities are endless. Go running for twenty minutes and see how good (if exhausted) you feel afterward. Check out www.nancyredd.com for a long list of other free activities to get yourself in tip-top shape. You'd be surprised how many calories these simple activities burn.

If you feel compelled to exercise in a workout-dedicated environment, become involved with your local 4-H club, community center (like a YWCA), or school's sports teams. Group athletics is a great way to make friends AND get in shape. Also, there may be neighborhood gyms or clubs that are free for students or that have special, affordable rates for young members. Also check with your school; it might have some fitness resources you can use as well.

Not only are there tons of cheap ways to get in shape, it's even possible to MAKE money losing weight. Start up a dog walking business or apply for a job (or maybe volunteer) to work with youth athletic teams. Running after children all afternoon is sure to burn some calories while making a difference in the kids' lives and perhaps putting some cash in your pocket. Interested in earning for others? Sign up for a walkathon and ask for charity donations for every mile you walk. Talk about great motivation!

**Diet.** As far as food is concerned, you don't have to follow a costly nutrition plan or load up on expensive health food items to eat better. Actually, cutting down on eating junk and candy and preparing yummy, healthy foods at home can help you lose weight and SAVE you money.

For example, some beverages not only have more calories than an entire meal but also cost as much as one! Don't believe me? What about that afternoon specialty coffee drink? It may be costing you nearly five bucks and seven hundred calories. Because it takes 3,500 extra calories to gain a pound, that coffee alone is a fifth of a pound! That same five dollars at the same shop could get you a hot tea with skim milk AND a yogurt cup, saving you five hundred calories (and maybe a heart attack).

Watching what you drink is a quick, easy, and cheap way to lose weight. Besides specialty coffees, fruit juices, milkshakes, and sugary sodas contain tons of calories. Just by cutting out your afternoon soda habit (or by switching to sugar-free), you save as much as two hundred calories a day. That might not sound like much at first, but added up, it equals over twenty pounds saved a year! So check the nutrition labels on the package or on

*fast fact*

*Are there certain foods that make you feel bloated, tired, and still hungry after you eat them? If so, you may have one of many potential food sensitivities, meaning that your body doesn't react well when you ingest certain things. If this happens to you, keep a food journal and try to pinpoint the problem. The most common food sensitivities are eggs, shellfish, milk, nuts, and soy.*

the product's Web site before chugging away. See the facing page for help understanding nutrition labels.

Also, stop snacking on junk! Just like coffee drinks, chips, candy, and other unhealthy snack foods can sneakily pack on pudge. If you must munch, instead of spending money at the vending machine, use that cash to buy fruits, vegetables, granola bars, yogurt, and other healthy items to keep in your bag so you can feel less tempted!

You may even want to try your hand at making your lunch or cooking meals at home. When channeling your inner Iron Chef, you have more control over what goes into your food, making it healthier and even tastier! For cheap, healthy recipes and for more ways to get fit frugally, check out www.nancyredd.com.

F.Y.I.

# PORTION CONTROL

We all know a healthy diet doesn't include jumbo fries or extra-large colas, but what ARE the right portion sizes for proper weight control? Here are some guidelines to get you started:

| FOOD | SERVING SIZE | WHAT A SERVING LOOKS LIKE |
|---|---|---|
| Bowl of cereal | I Cup | Balled-up fist |
| Pancake | I | Compact Disc |
| Meat, fish, or chicken | 3 ounces | Deck of cards |
| Peanut butter | 2 tablespoons | Golf ball |
| Cooking oil | I teaspoon | The tip of your thumb |
| Cheese | I.5 ounces | Lipstick tube |

Do those quantities surprise you? Yes, a serving of meat should be the size of a deck of cards, and a serving of cereal is the size of your fist. Still, when have you ever seen something that small in a restaurant? Portion sizes in restaurants are getting larger and larger, which is a big reason we're gaining weight! Try asking for a to-go container or see if a friend wants to split a dish with you. There's sure to be enough for two!

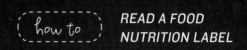

**Nutrition Facts**
Serving Size 8 fl oz (240mL)
Servings Per Container 2

100% Pure Squeezed Grapefru

INGREDIENTS: 100%
Squeezed Grapefru
*Contains juice fro

*how to*

## READ A FOOD NUTRITION LABEL

Ever wonder what all those numbers and percentages mean on your food packaging? While it's not rocket science, it can be a bit complicated to figure out. Never fear, here's a guide to help you get the most information possible about the food you eat.

The most important thing to look for on the nutrition label is the "Suggested Serving Size." ① While the outside of a box of twelve cookies might say a serving is only eighty calories, the suggested serving size may be only one cookie, meaning that when you eat three you're tripling your calories! Keep a close eye out for puny portions that might trick you into thinking you're eating fewer calories than you actually are. This one container has TWO servings listed, meaning that if you drink the whole thing, you're going to have to double the numbers—sneaky!

Next, take a look at the "Daily Reference Value" (DRV) ② column. This percentage tells how much of your daily allotment of fat, sugar, carbohydrates, fiber, and vitamins one serving of the food item contains. The Food and Drug Administration (FDA) has determined that a recommended daily total for a teenage girl or moderately-active woman is:

- 2,000 calories
- 300 grams of carbohydrates
- less than 65 grams of fat (less than 20 of these grams should be saturated fat)
- 50 grams of protein
- 25 grams of fiber
- less than 2,400 milligrams of sodium
- less than 300 milligrams of cholesterol

So, if the double cheeseburger you ate for lunch had 440 calories and 23 grams of fat (II grams being saturated fat), you ate only 22 percent of your daily calories, but you consumed 35 percent of your daily fat intake and 54 percent of your saturated fat intake. This means that to stay healthy you'll need to pick a much less fatty meal for dinner.

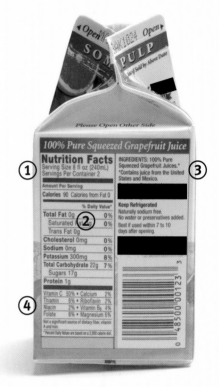

③ Ingredients. Labels list ingredients from most to least weight in the item. You might be surprised to see that the first ingredient in many foods is actually water! In this case nothing has been added, but in many juices, extra sugar has been added, ramping up the calorie and carbohydrate content.

④ Vitamins & Nutrients. Each label must share daily value percentages of calcium, iron, and vitamins A and C, though some food labels also include other listings. You should try to meet 100 percent of the daily value of these vitamins and nutrients every day.

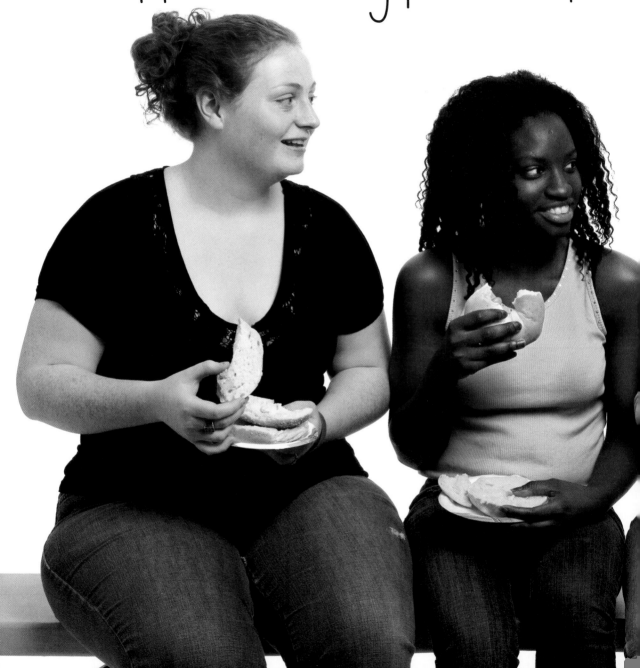

DRAMA #4

# I eat the same as my friends, but

# I'm the only one who gains weight.

## WHAT'S GOING ON?

*I pack on pounds from only one piece of pizza while my cousins can eat a whole pie each and not gain a thing. It's so not fair!*

Calories affect individuals differently because everyone's body processes calories at a different rate. It's called your metabolism. Your metabolism works off of your basal metabolic rate (BMR), the minimum number of calories your body needs to keep you alive, regardless of your physical activity. BMR supports such basic processes as breathing, breaking down food, and keeping your heart and brain working. If you were in a coma, you would need only enough calories to support your BMR, but in our everyday lives, we need a bunch of additional calories to keep us running and ripping through our hectic schedules. For example, reading this book takes more calories than sleeping, so to remain the same weight, you need to eat enough to give you the energy to get through it. Your metabolism slows down or speeds up, depending on a variety of factors.

*Four main ones are:*

- **age.** Older folks have a slower metabolism than younger people.

- **gender.** Men have faster metabolism rates than women do.

- **physical activity.** People who are physically active have faster metabolisms than those who sit around for most of their day.

- **diet.** People who don't eat enough or who eat unhealthily have slower metabolisms than people who have good eating habits.

215

So, it's safe to say that a teen boy will have a faster metabolism than a thirty-year-old woman, right? Not always, and especially not if that guy sits at his computer all day eating candy bars! While you can't do anything about your age or gender, your diet and physical activity both have a tremendous effect on your BMR.

If you eat healthily and have a lot of muscle, your body burns more calories, meaning you can eat more and not gain as much weight. Also, people who exercise often and have more muscle on their body have a higher BMR because muscle burns more calories than fat burns.

On the other hand, if you're not eating healthily (see page 211 for more information), or if you go long periods between meals, your body learns to conserve fuel, meaning it needs fewer calories to survive, causing you to gain weight more easily.

fast fact

*Are you feeling more sluggish or depressed than usual? Are you gaining weight but not eating any differently? The problem may lie in your thyroid, which is a gland in your neck that puts out hormones that control your metabolic rate. If it's working sluggishly, you may experience fatigue, weight gain, abnormal periods, dry skin, and more. If you suspect a thyroid problem, see your doctor as soon as possible. A physician can prescribe medicine to regulate your thyroid.*

## HOW DO I DEAL?

Contrary to popular belief, not many people really have a "slow metabolism." Some people naturally maintain a higher weight than others, but most of us just aren't caring for our bodies as well as we should.

Be honest: What are your habits? Before blaming your bulges on your body's genetics, take note of your daily schedule. Skipping meals, eating too late in the evening, and not eating enough calories all slow down your metabolism, making the maintenance of a healthy weight more difficult.

To jumpstart your metabolic engine, make sure to eat a good breakfast and eat small, healthy snacks during the day, cutting out the junk food. Your metabolism naturally slows down in the evening, so try to have your dinner at least three hours before bedtime.

Another way to get your body to speed up is exercise. A fitness routine will build calorie-burning muscle, and send your metabolism up, up, UP!

Make sure you're not comparing your normal, healthy body to the ones you see on television or magazines. Chances are, it's not their metabolism that keeps the weight off but an artist who specializes in photographic airbrushing (see page 240 for more). If you still feel as if food reacts differently with you than others, the problem might by your thyroid (see the fast fact, above).

# THE PROPER WAY TO CRUNCH

A tight tummy looks great, and crunches build metabolism-boosting stomach muscles. You can do this exercise anywhere.

Make sure you reach for those six-pack abs the right way. Done improperly, abdominal exercises are not effective and can hurt your neck and back.

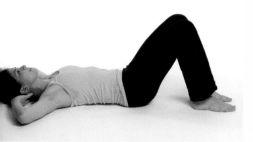

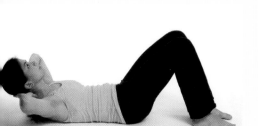

*Follow these steps to keep from wasting time and risking injury:*

1. Lie down on the floor with your hands behind your neck and your feet flat on the floor about a foot away from your rear. Bend your knees and align your heels with your hips.

2. When you're ready to crunch, keep your head parallel to the floor and your eyes staring up at the ceiling. DO NOT PULL on your neck. Let your stomach do the work as you slowly lift your shoulders up to about a 30-degree angle. Rising beyond that doesn't work the muscles properly and might injure your back.

3. Squeeze and hold for three seconds, then slowly return your shoulders to the floor.

4. Repeat at least ten times at first, working your way up to more as you get stronger.

---

### *SIGNS YOU'RE NOT CRUNCHING CORRECTLY*

**Your neck hurts.** This means you're using your hands—not your stomach—to pull yourself up. To make the crunch easier on you (and your neck), fold your arms across your chest when you lift.

**You're going quickly.** Going too fast doesn't allow enough time for your muscles to feel the burn every crunch. Aim for smooth, controlled motions—no bouncing!

**It's too easy.** If you don't feel your muscles working in your stomach, you're probably pulling yourself up with your arms and not your abdominal muscles.

I'll never be thin enough.

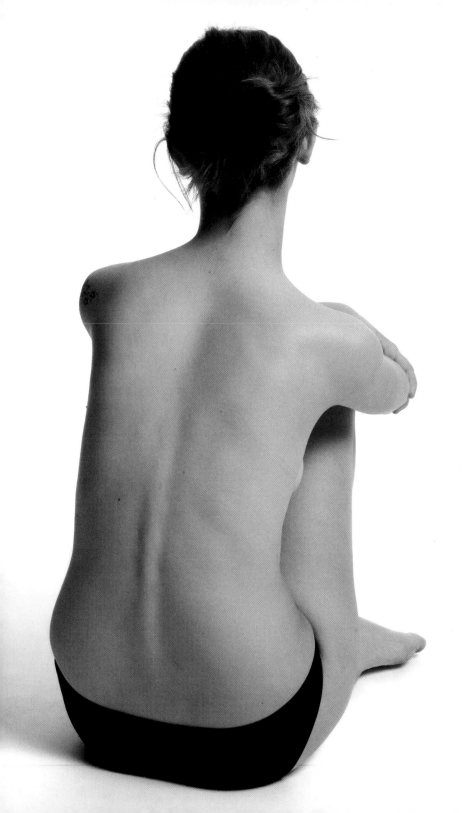

## WHAT'S GOING ON?

*Mirror, mirror, on the wall, who's the thinnest of them all?*

If you catch yourself asking that question and answering, "I wish ME!" then you might be caught up in a dangerous rat race to the thinnest line.

Most Americans are getting fatter and fatter. Still, a surprising number—nearly 5 percent of eighteen to twenty-four-year-olds—are actually UNDERweight. Being extremely thin and underweight is often promoted in the media as more attractive and desirable. Sad, but true.

Ultrathin beauty ideals are not only unfair, but also unrealistic. The average American woman is actually five feet four inches tall and weighs 163 pounds. Most runway models stand five feet ten or five feet eleven inches tall. They average 120 to 124 pounds. While some women are naturally slim, lots, if not most, of those ultra-thin bodies get that way through extreme dieting and compulsive exercise.

Are you constantly on a diet, always working to improve your body, and never fully satisfied with the results, no matter what? If so, you're not the only one. It's estimated that an amazing 63 percent of teenage girls use "unhealthy" methods to control their weight, with over 20 percent using "very unhealthy" methods such as diuretics (water pills), diet pills, vomiting, laxatives, and skipping meals altogether.

## F.Y.I.

# DIETING CAN MAKE YOU GAIN WEIGHT

Teens who diet are over THREE TIMES more likely to be overweight in their twenties. Why? Many factors contribute, but it's mostly because eating too little for an extended period of time starves your body into survival mode, ruining your metabolism (see page 215 for more about metabolism). When food is consumed by a healthy person with a normal metabolism, the body tries to use as many of the calories as possible as quickly as it can. In someone who has not been eating enough for an extended period of time, the body's metabolism becomes "afraid" of not getting enough to survive, and it slows down in an attempt to store as many calories as possible for the future. Unfortunately, even after you begin eating a normal amount, your body might never again "believe" that it's safe to behave properly. So, denying your body might make you thinner now, but your bad habits will make keeping your weight down later very difficult.

Do you think you'll never be thin enough? Is your weight below normal on the BMI chart on page 202? How far are you going in your search for slimness? Can you stop this unhealthy cycle?

If not, it's possible that you may be suffering from an eating disorder.

Eating disorders are so complicated that each one of them could fill a whole book (and many of them do!). They all have emotional, physical, and environmental causes that combine in ways that are as unique as we are. There are common symptoms and long-term consequences for each disorder, but every individual is not going to have the same experience. Many people suffer from more than one disorder at a time, and respond in different ways to different treatments.

It's impossible to generalize about eating disorders and to cover them accurately in two or three sentences, but the following information may help you identify a problem that is bothering you. Check out some of the resources on page 256 for complete, reliable, and up-to-date information from trustworthy Web sites and professionals who research and treat these specific conditions.

*fast fact*

*A related struggle that many of girls face is compulsive or extreme exercising. Are you obsessed with the gym? Do you get upset if you haven't burned a certain number of calories each day? Do you feel obligated to work out through pain, fatigue, and hunger? Also known as anorexia athletica or exercise bulimia, compulsive exercising can be just as dangerous as bulimia or anorexia, and it often goes hand in hand with eating disorders.*

### ANOREXIA

Anorexics effectively starve themselves; they can never be thin enough. In addition to extreme weight loss, anorexia can stop your period, make you cold all the time, throw off your metabolism forever, and cause fine hair to grow all over your body and face. Anorexia can land you in the hospital with a heart attack or liver and kidney damage. These and other serious complications, if left untreated for too long, can kill you—as it has famous models and athletes. Roughly 10 percent of diagnosed anorexics die.

### BULIMIA

Bulimics binge on a lot of food (see binge eating) and then purge their body of the food by vomiting or using laxatives. A person with bulimia may be thin, normal weight, or overweight. Bulimia can cause dry lips and skin, eroded teeth (from stomach acids eating the enamel away), broken blood vessels around the eyes, ripping of the esophagus (from the strain of purging), a permanently damaged metabolism, liver and kidney damage, a weakened heart, and other severe complications, including death. Studies indicate that by their first year of college, over 4 percent of young women have a history of bulimia. Some sources think that number is as high as 18 percent.

### BINGE EATING

Binge eaters go on food "binges" when they gorge themselves on tons of food until they cannot eat any more. Sometimes, they deliberately purge (making them bulimic), but many binge eaters do not rid themselves of the food. Because of the constant extra calories, unless they are extreme dieters or compulsive exercisers, many binge eaters are overweight or obese. Around 3 percent of women suffer from binge eating disorder, making it more prevalent than anorexia and almost as common as bulimia.

### COMPULSIVE OVEREATING

Compulsive overeaters are addicted to food. No amount of food or frequency of meals is satisfying, as eating is not just about feeling full physically. Overeating is usually an attempt to fill an emotional hunger. The compulsive overeater chows down when she is stressed, nervous, lonely, excited, bored . . . any change in emotion can be an excuse to eat. Overeaters are usually overweight or obese, and it is just as hard for an overeater to stop eating too much as it is for an anorexic to eat enough.

## HOW DO I DEAL?

Do any of these descriptions hit home with you, even just a little bit? If so, no matter how hard it is to admit it, you must seek help NOW. If caught early, eating disorders and their complications are treatable, but if you don't get help soon enough, the problem can quickly spiral out of control and cause permanent damage. In addition to ruining your metabolism, complications from long-term eating disorders can include paralysis, bone disorders, tooth decay, heart problems, infertility, and DEATH.

If you have an eating disorder, DON'T BE ASHAMED. Millions of young women (upwards of ten million!) are in the same position as you. Because of shame, many do not seek help. It might be scary and embarrassing to admit your issues, but you should feel proud of yourself for taking control of your body, your mind, and your health.

When looking for help, your doctor is a safe place to start. *Ask your doctor* to recommend you to someone who specializes in eating disorders. If the doctor or a specialist is not available for you to confide in, any trusted adult is fine—as long as you don't put it off! If you want to speak to someone anonymously first, call the National Eating Disorders Association's hotline at 1-800-931-2237. Chances are good you'll get someone on the line who knows from personal experience what you're talking about and how you're feeling. As mentioned earlier, check the resources section in the back of this book for other safe and reliable assistance. There is a lot of support out there—and a LOT of hope.

# DIE-T PILLS

Just because you can purchase many weight-loss supplements without a prescription doesn't make them safe. A lot of over-the-counter pills and medicines that promise to quickly shed pounds or suppress your appetite contain dangerous ingredients that can seriously damage your health and even kill. Even ones labeled "all-natural" can be hazardous to your health.

Some common side effects from weight-loss supplements include increased heart rate and irregular heartbeats, high blood pressure, headaches and dizziness, insomnia (inability to sleep), anxiety and nervousness, and depression.

Because weight-loss supplements aren't carefully regulated in the way that food and other medicines are, most of these dangerous supplements don't even work, meaning you might be risking your life for nothing! Also, because there are no regulations, an unsafe product may not be removed from shelves until a number of people have suffered serious health problems or even DIED from taking it!

Don't buy into this billion dollar a year industry. Protect yourself and your health by turning to page 210 for tips on getting in shape the right way.

DRAMA #6

# I'm depressed.

## WHAT'S GOING ON?

Sometimes body drama isn't just physical. Let's face it—at times, life sucks. We all experience sadness, shame, self-hate, anger, anxiety, frustration, negativity, and hopelessness at various times and for a variety of reasons. A bad grade or a huge pimple might have us moping around for a bit, while breaking up with a romantic partner might keep us down for a couple of weeks! Other times we might just wake up on the wrong side of the bed or have a bad day. It's usually easy for us to get back to our "normal" selves in a few days, but sometimes these feelings consume us for extended periods of time, affecting our entire lives and how we feel about ourselves. This experience is commonly referred to as depression.

Feel like you might be depressed? See if you recognize any of these symptoms.

*For more than two weeks at a time, have you ever found yourself*
- becoming more easily frustrated, angered, moody, irritable, combative, or disturbed?
- having more difficulty than usual focusing in school or elsewhere?
- thinking about or actually hurting yourself?
- thinking frequently about death or killing yourself?
- avoiding hanging out with or talking to your friends and family?
- taking less care of yourself and your health?
- changing your eating habits to eating either much more or much less than usual?
- changing your sleeping habits to sleeping either much more or much less than usual?
- being unable to shake constant feelings of hopelessness, sadness, despair?
- constantly losing your temper and being rude to others?
- enjoying yourself or your life less than usual?

If any of these warning signs sound familiar to you, you're not alone. About 20 percent of American teenagers have experienced one or more bouts of depression. Although it's easy to brush off depression as crankiness or having a bad attitude, it's actually a serious medical condition that requires professional help to conquer.

*There are many reasons you might be depressed. Some common ones include:*

- **stress.** Tremendous amounts of pressure from family, friends, relationships, and school (not to mention society) can trigger depression.
- **hormones.** Fluctuating levels of hormones can greatly affect our emotions, triggering periods of depression.
- **brain chemistry.** Chemical imbalances in the brain frequently cause depression.
- **genetics.** While clinical depression can happen to anyone, it often occurs in individuals who have a parent, sibling, or other family member who has suffered from depression as well.

*Oftentimes, depression is brought on by traumatic things that happen to us such as:*

- the illness or death of someone close to you
- family issues, such as your parents, siblings, or close relatives dealing with substance abuse, money troubles, violence, or divorce
- personal issues, such as illness, substance abuse, or an eating disorder (see page 220 for more information)
- experiencing or witnessing emotional abuse, physical abuse, or sexual assault (see page 230 for more information on handling assault)

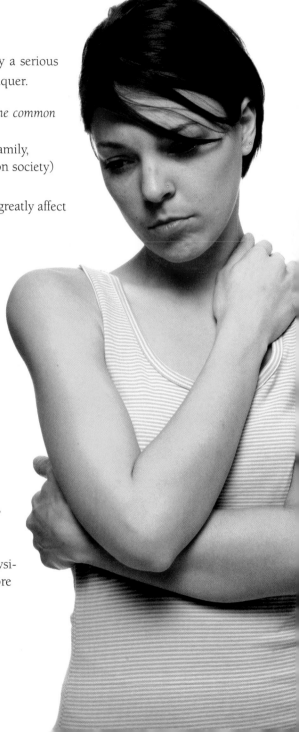

There are various types and levels of depression. Major depression doesn't just bring your mood down—it affects your entire life! You might find yourself unable to enjoy activities that you normally love, and your schoolwork, your relationships with friends and family, and even your eating and sleeping patterns may suffer tremendously. With major depression, you might have periods of time where you are completely dysfunctional (a fancy way of saying unable to do hardly anything at all) for weeks or months at a time. Sadly, you might have frequent thoughts of hurting yourself, including suicide.

☼ **CAUTION: If you have ANY thoughts of hurting or killing yourself, another person, or an animal, you MUST seek help IMMEDIATELY.**

Don't think that your life has to be completely upside-down for you to be diagnosed as depressed. If you're constantly feeling down and are unable to shake your negative feelings, even if you don't fully recognize yourself in the warning signs, your doctor or therapist might diagnose you with some level of depression. Or, upon examination, your doctor might notice symptoms of other medical conditions that affect your mood and behavior or that cause depression as a side effect. For example, some medications taken for physical conditions cause depressionlike symptoms. However, only a trained professional can make this distinction.

## HOW DO I DEAL?

Think you might suffer from depression? First things first: YOU ARE NOT CRAZY! Depression doesn't come about because of something you did, nor does it mean that there's something wrong with your character or personality.

What it does mean is that you cannot remain quiet about what's going on. Don't try to push away the awareness that you might have a medical condition. Remember: Depression usually doesn't just "go away," so don't try to just snap out of it. _See your doctor immediately_ to start treatment. A doctor, therapist, or other trained professional can make you feel much better because he or she will

- listen to you and your concerns with a knowledgeable and understanding ear;
- record and monitor your moods to track your progress in getting better;
- refer you to a therapist or a specialist who can help you even more; and
- (perhaps) prescribe medication.

For information on how to find professional help, see the resources on page 256 and get started on the road to feeling better ASAP.

If you don't think that you are seriously depressed but you still feel really down or blue, or if something else is emotionally or mentally bothering you, there's no harm in seeking help or talking to someone about your problems. Sometimes, getting concerns off your chest early will prevent them from ballooning into larger, more painful issues. Your school counselor or another trusted adult might be a good starting point. By working through your anxieties now, you could be preventing depression down the road.

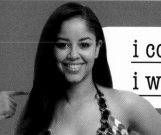

## i confess:
## i went to therapy.

My junior year in college I won $250,000 on *Who Wants to Be a Millionaire?*—an unusual experience for anyone, especially a college kid, and I ended up a total wreck. Everyone expected me to be on top of the world, but the stress and excitement were too much for a twenty-year-old to handle. I couldn't sleep and my hair was falling out. I had gained back all the weight I had lost in high school, people who were close to me started being mean for no reason, and I was being hit up for money by strangers AND family members, even after I'd given much of it away! I had no one to talk to, so after seeing a flyer on campus advertising free counseling, I made an appointment and poured out my problems to a therapist, who gave me wonderful advice and taught me new ways to handle stress. I could yell, complain, and say all the things I wanted to without anyone else knowing! It was just what I needed, and it made a big difference.

We all go through rough times in our lives, and talking things out with a professional is the best way to avoid turning an issue now into bigger problems later on. There's no shame in seeking help for your problems, and there are many people in your life who can help. Do you have a favorite teacher, school counselor, principal, or nurse you can confide in? Whomever you choose, sharing your feelings and getting insight and support from a professional is important. I know from experience!

# I'm harming my body.

## WHAT'S GOING ON?

*Girls—be pretty. Be popular. Be pleasant. Be PERFECT! Oh, and while you're at it, DON'T get in trouble, DON'T have a bad attitude, DON'T do drugs or drink, and DON'T get pregnant. DON'T. MAKE. ANY. MISTAKES. EVER! Got that?*

In general, society earmarks us girls as the more polite sex, more studious, more patient, and better at adjusting to different environments than men. Women are SO responsible that, naturally, we take better care of ourselves and our bodies, right?

Oftentimes, the answer is no.

In trying to cope with difficult pressure, overwhelming stress, and intense feelings, sometimes we make extremely unhealthy decisions about how to treat and take care of our bodies. The choices we make in attempts to stifle feelings of self-hate, loss, rage, hopelessness, depression, shame, anxiety, and other emotions often actually hurt us even more. In an attempt to feel better, people sometimes harm themselves by abusing alcohol, drugs, and other substances (see facing page). Eating disorders (see page 220) are often brought on by painful feelings and emotions as well.

Another very harmful way some teens try to cope is self-injury, which is the act of purposefully physically harming oneself.

*People who self-injure choose different ways to hurt themselves:*
- cutting their skin with a knife or other sharp object
- burning, poking, or hitting themselves
- pulling, tweezing, or tearing out their own hair (see page 185 for more information on trichotillomania)
- bruising themselves or breaking their own bones

It's hard to determine exactly how many girls in America are injuring themselves because many are too ashamed to admit what they are doing and to seek help; some experts think that it is the fastest rising issue for teen girls. In England, it was recently found that about 11 percent of fif-teen- to sixteen-year-old girls reported a deliberate act of self-injury.

## HOW DO I DEAL?

*Do you*

- cut, scratch, or cause yourself harm on purpose?
- feel "better" or relieved after hurting yourself?
- find yourself craving the feeling you get when you're injuring yourself?
- have to hide scars from self-attacks?

If you see yourself in these descriptions you probably already know something's wrong, but you may not know what to do about it. You are not alone, and it is not your fault. *You need professional advice, therapy, support, determination, and perhaps medication IMMEDIATELY.* Don't try to fix your problems on your own. Your doctor or a counselor is the best place to begin seeking help. Turn to page 250 to find a professional who will help you get started on the road to recovery today. There is a lot of sup-port out there to help you heal emotionally as well as physically, so DON'T GIVE UP HOPE!

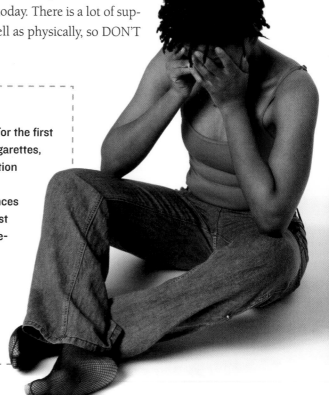

### ALCOHOL AND SUBSTANCE ABUSE

Self-injury isn't the only way we hurt ourselves. For the first time in history, girls are now starting to smoke cigarettes, use marijuana, drink alcohol, and abuse prescription drugs at higher rates than boys.

Are you addicted to alcohol or other substances and need them in order to relax, calm down, or just because? Are you doing drugs or drinking on a fre-quent basis? Can you not stop?

GET HELP NOW. The earlier you seek help, the more easily you can quit. Check out www .nancyredd.com and the substance abuse re-sources on page 256 for more information on how to find help.

# WHEN SOMEONE ELSE HARMS YOUR BODY

NO ONE, AND I MEAN NO ONE, HAS THE RIGHT TO HURT YOUR BODY. Unfortunately, as women we are more vulnerable to physical harm than men are, but that doesn't mean we are powerless to protect ourselves. As scary as speaking out about such matters may seem, you DO have the courage to stand up and speak out, and there ARE safe places you can go.

## PHYSICAL ASSAULT

In the United States, more than 1.4 million teenagers are physically assaulted each year. If you are physically assaulted, call The National Center for Victims of Crime, which has a hotline available (Monday through Friday from 8:30 A.M. to 8:30 P.M. EST): 1-800-FYI-CALL. It's staffed with people who can talk confidentially about your concerns and can give you advice on reporting your assailant. You can also call the Teen Relationship National Hotline at 1-800-799-SAFE for help anytime.

## SEXUAL ASSAULT

**Rape.** Rape is defined as the forced penetration of one's body orally, vaginally, or anally. Sadly, people between the ages of twelve and nineteen make up the largest percentage of rape victims. Nearly three-fourths of rapes are committed by someone the victim knows, with 28 percent of the crimes committed by a former sex partner or relative (see below for more information on incest). Although the number of rapes has fallen in recent years, the act of rape still occurs *once every eight minutes.* More than half of sexual assaults go unreported, sometimes because of fear or shame, but often because the victim doesn't know what to do.

**Incest.** For many young women, sexual assault hits extremely close to home. Many sexual assaults are by family members, making the victims sufferers of incest. Being related to your attacker is no reason to keep the assault a secret. You might feel torn because this person is someone you love and depend on, and the relative might threaten you or make you feel guilty, but remember this: Incest is a crime. It is never a family member's right to assault you, no matter what he (or she) says. If you have any type of interaction with a relative that makes you feel uncomfortable, TELL SOMEONE. This is YOUR body and YOUR life. You deserve to live in a home (and body) that is free from fear.

**Other kinds of sexual assault.** Rape isn't the only type of sexual assault. ANY unwanted physical touch (fondling, kissing, or rubbing against your body) or unwanted verbal or visual exchange (such as calling you suggestive names or giving you pornography) is considered sexual assault and MUST be taken SERIOUSLY. Nearly three-fourths of all sexual assaults are committed by someone the victim knows well.

### If you are raped, it's important to follow these steps:

**Get to a safe place.** A hospital is the best place to go first. Tell the emergency room personnel your situation and they'll know how to help you. The hospital can give you medications to ward off sexually transmitted infections and prevent pregnancy. If there aren't any hospitals around, the next best location is a police station, and don't worry if you don't have any money for transportation. The hospital or police station will pay for the cab once you arrive and explain your situation. If a cab is not available, call 911 from the nearest pay phone or convenience store and request a police car or ambulance to take you to the hospital.

**Do not bathe or change clothes.** As awful and gross as you might feel after an assault, your body might be holding the only evidence that can put your attacker behind bars. The hospital will take care of you and protect your rights and the evidence. It's understandable why you might not want to follow this step, due to feeling shameful about the sexual assault. Waiting until later to shower and allowing the hospital to confidentially retain evidence, however, makes conviction more likely if your assailant goes to trial.

Being violated is a very serious matter, and your mind can be your worst enemy when your body is trying to heal. The Rape, Abuse, & Incest National Network has a confidential 24/7 helpline (1-800-656-HOPE) and an online hotline at www.rainn.org. Or, you can speak with a doctor, nurse, or your school counselor about setting you up to talk with a professional who specializes in helping victims of rape.

Because of the emotional fallout involved, getting immediate help for any type of assault is critical. Your doctor, school counselor, or other professional (see right) can help you work through this experience and can also protect you from future assault. A warning: Victims often suffer from depression, turn to alcohol and drugs, or think about suicide. I can't say this enough: Get help and support IMMEDIATELY.

## YOU ARE NOT ALONE.

### A WORD ABOUT PROFESSIONAL HELP

If you need or want assistance for any reason, many different people can offer professional help and support. Professionals you might seek out include psychiatrists, psychologists, social workers, counselors, therapists, medical doctors, or nurses. Whatever they're called, these professionals are there to help you. They will talk with you, sometimes prescribe medication, or simply point you toward the right person to get you all the help you need. Keep in mind that sometimes the people we confide in don't always take us seriously the first time we say we have an issue. If you don't find what you're looking for in the first person you ask, don't give up. KEEP TRYING until you get the help you need and deserve.

DRAMA #8 I'm obsessed with my looks.

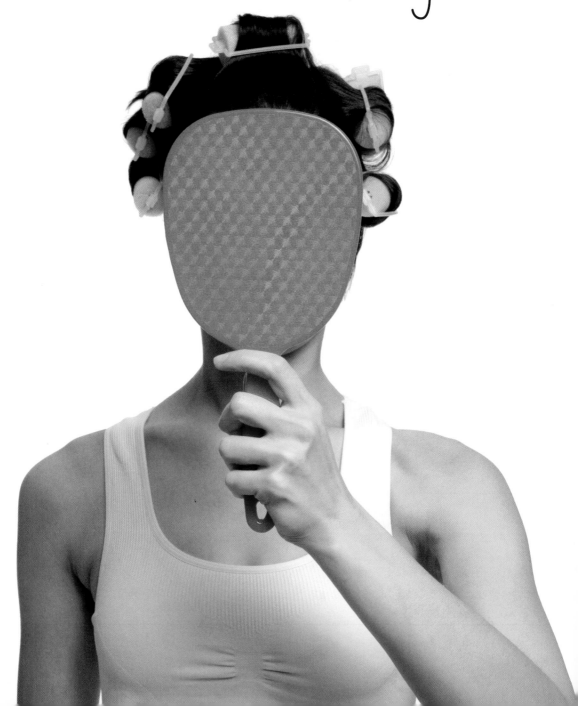

## WHAT'S GOING ON?

*No, for the last time, that dress does not make your hips look too wide!*

Is primping taking so much of your time that life seems to be passing you by? Does your everyday routine always make you late for class because you stare into your closet for hours, change outfits dozens of times, and take forever to find something that you don't hate? Do you check the mirror every five minutes to make sure everything's in perfect order? Are you never satisfied with how you look?

Are you still reading this? Are you nodding your head? Because if you are, then you may be over-the-top-obsessed with the way you look!

It's incredible how much time and energy we spend thinking about things that don't matter much—or at all—in the grand scheme of your life. Everyone, to an extent, worries about keeping up appearances, and of course we all want to look our best. Sometimes, anxiety about fitting in, feeling attractive, and finding friends can cause us to go too far. While there is an actual body obsession disorder that some people suffer from (see Body Dysmorphic Disorder below), most of us who obsess are just huge worrywarts when it comes to how we look and, of course, how other people think we look. Problem is, even though much of the effort you put into this superficiality is for others, it's easy to come across as a self-absorbed drama queen.

# BODY DYSMORPHIC DISORDER

Sometimes, being worried about how we look is more than just a desire to look good—it's a disorder. Normal-looking, healthy women who suffer from Body Dysmorphic Disorder (BDD) obsess over their body drama to an unhealthy degree, thinking themselves unattractive or even disfigured. BDD sufferers spend hours each day thinking about and trying to conceal their flaws. Often, the perceived imperfection is small and unnoticeable to others—from a weird arm freckle, to a slightly crooked earlobe, to one eye being wider than the other.

Many women with BDD are simply written off as having normal anxieties so they don't get help, but there are small differences between people with BDD and "regular" worrying are obvious to a professional. If your appearance is causing you concern beyond the superficial, *see your doctor*. If your doctor brushes you off, insist on getting a referral to an experienced professional who will take you seriously.

## HOW DO I DEAL?

Transitioning from a got-it-all-together glamour-puss to a regular girl isn't always easy. If you'd like to try spending more time on your life than your looks, a good way to start toning down your daily quests for perfection is by setting some boundaries. Try to give yourself a time limit for how much energy you'll spend on beautification and obsession each day. Stick to that limit!

Don't try to quit primping cold turkey, however. Taking care of yourself and your appearance, when it doesn't interfere with the rest of your life and the appropriate amount of time is spent, is healthy. Also, special occasions and important events are great opportunities to go "all out" and pay close attention to every detail.

Once you free yourself from time and emotion-consuming beauty routines every single day, however, you'll realize how many wonderful things there are to do besides worry about appearances. It's liberating to share yourself—your real self—with the world! As you spend more time on improving the real you rather than your hairdo, your friends might be shocked at first, but you may also be surprised by the positive feedback you get. As you get more comfortable in your own naturally beautiful skin, your friends will be more comfortable around you, too.

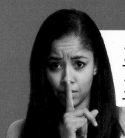

# i confess:
# i had to scale back.

I can't stand scales. Having been really heavy and really skinny, I never know how to trust that number. What is the weight I should be? Is that right? What if it's not the weight that I WANT to be?

While writing this book, I fluctuated between the weights of 155 to 132 pounds, depending upon how stressed I became (my Krispy Kreme phase was my heaviest) or how healthy I tried to be (for a few weeks I went to the gym every day). Regardless of how actively I was trying to stay in shape, I still felt the need to jump on the scales every single day. It felt like torture as the numbers whirled and came to an abrupt stop on that day's count. If it was less than yesterday, I cheered. If more, I sulked.

Except for that short-lived doughnut obsession, which gave new meaning to the phrase "a moment on the lips, a lifetime on the hips," according to the BMI chart, I remained within the "healthy" range for my height (five feet five).

Still, the scales drove me crazy! I kept checking the numbers, even although common sense told me that weight would fluctuate a pound or two (or even five) depending upon how much salt I had in my system, whether I had used the bathroom, and when I'd eaten my last meal.

Finally (luckily), it happened. My brother stole my scale. Calling me a hypocrite because of the messages I send in this book, he decided to take it upon himself to break my destructive scale cycle.

A scale-free month or so flew by, but when walking in the mall, I couldn't resist a twenty-five-cent scale in front of a fitness center. I popped in a quarter and held my breath. In the month that I'd stopped stressing out so much about my weight, I lost five pounds! The only thing I'd done differently was to worry less about my weight.

Fitness experts say not to weigh more than once a week, preferably once a month. After my experience, I'm in total agreement. By constantly obsessing, you're not giving yourself and your body a chance to regulate. If you're a scale addict like I was, take this moment right now and decide to stay scale-free for at least a week. See how much less stressed you'll feel!

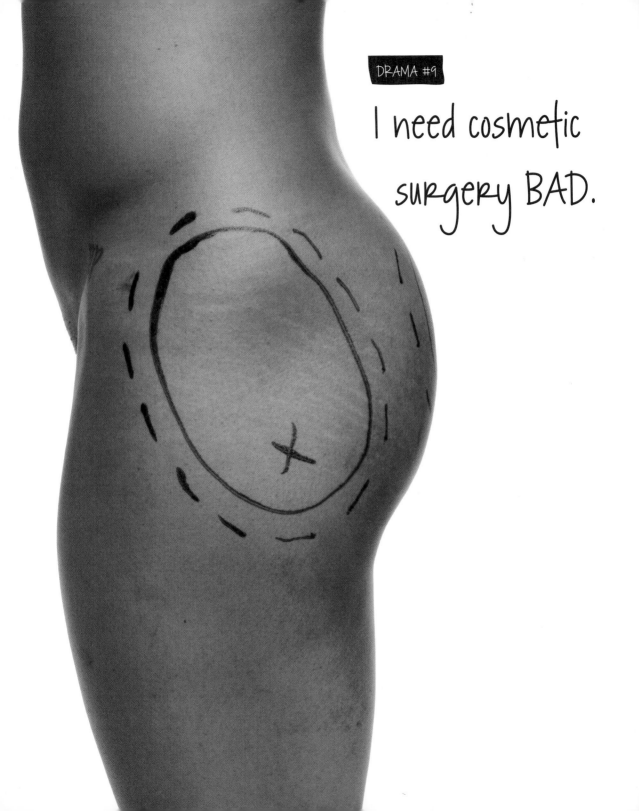

# NO, YOU DON'T.

## WHAT'S GOING ON?

If only your nose were straighter or your breasts larger or your toes shorter or your lips bigger, then life would be better and all your problems would go away, right? WRONG. If only life were that easy!

In reality, cosmetic surgery won't fix anything except what's on the outside. The same body issues you're dealing with inside will remain.

Television and magazines make cosmetic surgery seem the best and easiest way to improve our lives instantly, and celebrities often flaunt their cosmetic work as glamorous additions to their mystique.

☀ **CAUTION:** *The bottom line to cosmetic surgery is that it's*
- **expensive.** You could buy a car for the price of a new nose and boobs!
- **painful.** The pain won't necessarily end after surgery. Many patients complain about constant pain for years afterward.
- **risky.** All sorts of complications, including infections, chronic illnesses, and serious scarring, can occur. See "Nip and Tuck Nightmares," next page, for more details.
- **uncertain.** There are no guarantees. You could get your nose done and hate it even more than before.

Shockingly, despite these negatives, more than 300,000 cosmetic procedures are performed on people ages eighteen or younger each year. Recent estimates say that doctors annually perform about 48,000 nose jobs on teens, and they reshape the ears of almost 14,000. Nearly 4,000 teens get breast implants each year!

So you're not alone in your wish for wider lips or smaller hips, but that doesn't make your desire healthy or a good idea to act upon.

## HOW DO I DEAL?

The best advice is to WAIT, and not even for the reasons you might think. Most important is your LONG-TERM appearance. Your body doesn't really finish growing until you're around twenty-one years old, so if you have surgery on a pubescent nose or teenage boob, the body part might look completely out of whack after a big, unexpected growth spurt. While your doctor should know better, it's obvious from the statistics that some professionals aren't taking this important factor into consideration. So the responsibility is yours. Remember, cosmetic surgery is as serious as it gets. It's surgery, not a spa treatment, and there are serious risks involved. For example, in every 5,224 liposuction surgeries, one individual *dies*.

# NIP AND TUCK NIGHTMARES

A dent in your budget might not be the only damage done by cosmetic surgery. Some common plastic surgery complications include

- **skin death.** Medically known as necrosis (nuh-KROH-sis), sometimes the skin around surgical wounds dies, creating larger sores and causing scarring.

- **unevenness.** It's difficult to achieve perfect symmetry in plastic surgery, making it common to have one enhanced breast that is larger or higher, one liposuctioned thigh that is bigger, or, after a nose job, one nostril that is wider then the other.

- **numbness or tingling.** Surgical incisions may damage nerves, creating a constant tingling or a loss of sensation.

- **slow healing.** Surgery puts the body through a lot of trauma, and some people take longer to heal than others. It can take weeks, even months, for the body to recover from cosmetic surgery!

- **body dents.** Scarring and improper surgical procedures can create puckers, pockets, dimples, and other body imperfections that, once created, are often difficult or impossible to correct.

## WHAT IF THEY NOTICE?

Many times the real reason we want cosmetic surgery is because we think other people would like us more if we got it. Do you really have a problem with your ears, or are you just upset because your crush said something mean about them?

Don't let other people make your decisions for you. If, after careful thought, you think you can't deal with your body as it is for the next eighty years, *consult first with your own doctor.* But if you've thought long and hard and realized that you want a nose job or breast implants only because it seems as if everybody else is getting them, then chill out, save your money, and continue reading. With luck, some of this book's positive body self-esteem vibes will send your surgical dreams packing!

*This woman got liposuction fifteen years ago when she was a size two! Subsequent weight gain left her with lumps and indentations around her body, which she has tried to cover up with tattoos. She wishes she had exercised and eaten healthily instead of going under the knife.*

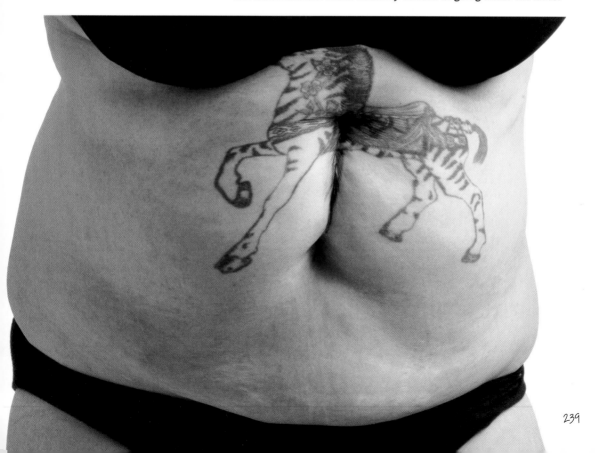

# THE **TRUTH** ABOUT **PHOTOS**

Whether we're driving down a billboard-plastered highway, flipping through gossip rags, Goo-gling our favorite musicians, or shopping online, photos are EVERYWHERE! Although the smooth-skinned, super-skinny bodies you see selling everything from clothing to cars appear to be real, they actually aren't. Unlike the women in this book, the pictures of bodies in magazines, ads, and even what you see when surfing the Internet, are usually heavily altered.

The media industry goes to great lengths to ensure that the models on their magazine covers (and on TV, in videos, on billboards and more) look thin, unblemished, and silky smooth. Many models spend thousands of dollars on beauty treatments and cosmetic surgery and are then pho-tographed and videoed under strategic lighting with an artist "touching up" the images afterward to ensure "perfection." Most of us aren't aware of how different these people would look if you actually met them on the street.

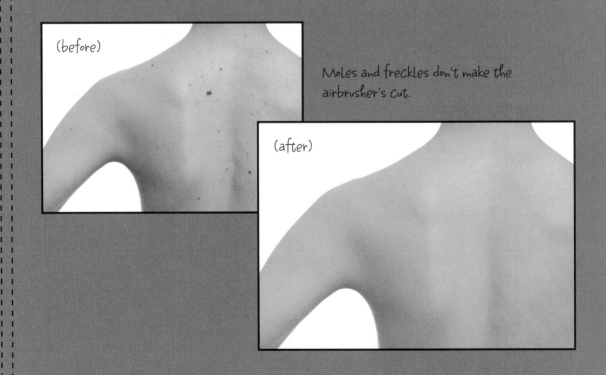

(before)

(after)

Moles and freckles don't make the airbrusher's cut.

(before)

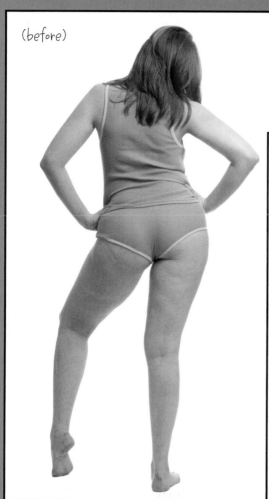

(after)

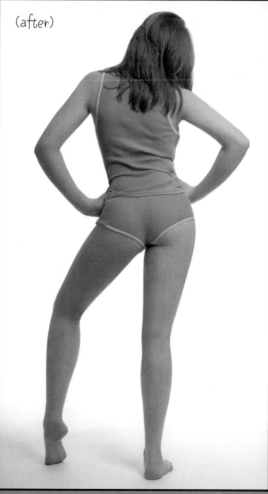

Airbrushers can shrink a healthy,
curvy size eight down to a stick.

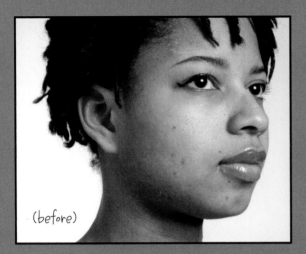

(before)

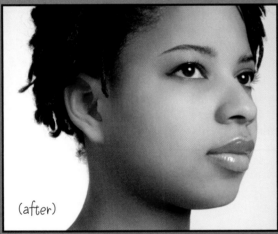

(after)

Airbrushers erase pimples and stray hairs in seconds.

Advances in computer software have made photo alteration easier (and scarier!) than ever. To show you how extreme this alteration process can be, we gave a digital artist who specializes in magazine airbrushing a few photos taken of the girls featured in this book and asked him to "fix" them as he would for an advertisement. As you can see on these pages, it's incredible how different a body can look after some careful computer modification.

It's so important to recognize the difference between real life and fantasy. The more you know about the alterations and enhancements that professionals use, the more ridiculous the whole obsession with fake perfection becomes. Now that you know the truth about how photos are altered, you can stop comparing your own body to the women you see on paper and feel much better about your own, one-of-a-kind shape.

Computer-generated boobs
and a smooth ponytail can be
created in just a few clicks!

(after)

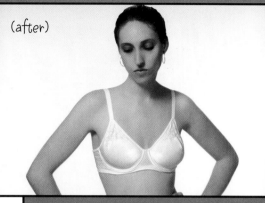

(before)

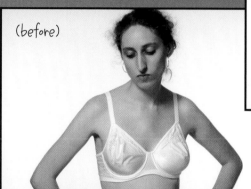

(before)

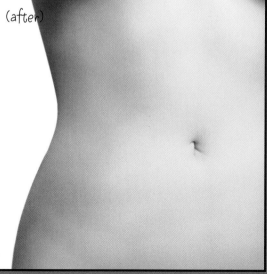

Stomachs shrink and pubic hairs don't
exist in magazineland.

(after)

# THE **TRUTH** ABOUT **BEAUTY**

From freckles to a flat butt to kinky hair to nearly K-cup chests, from completely bare down there to covered with hair *everywhere*, all of the artists, students, teachers, and other young women who were photographed for this book are *fabulous* in their natural, unaltered state, body drama and all—*just like you!* They're not supermodels, but they're super *role* models who dared to bare it all so you can know what *real* beauty looks like.

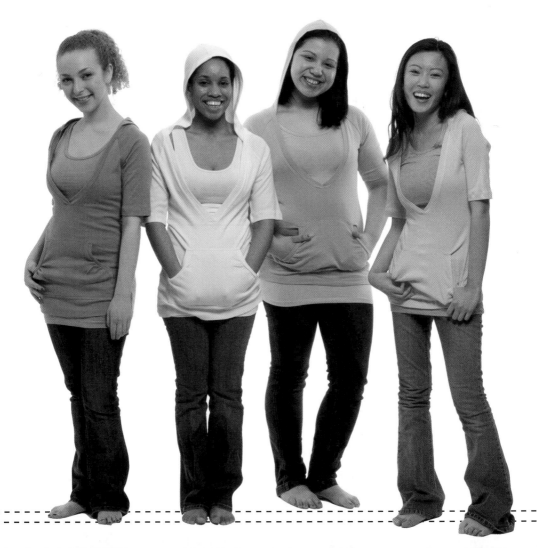

NO BODY'S PERFECT.

EVERY BODY
IS
BEAUTIFUL.

EVERY BODY'S DIFFERENT.

DIFFERENT IS BEAUTIFUL.

*Turn the page and see for yourself!*

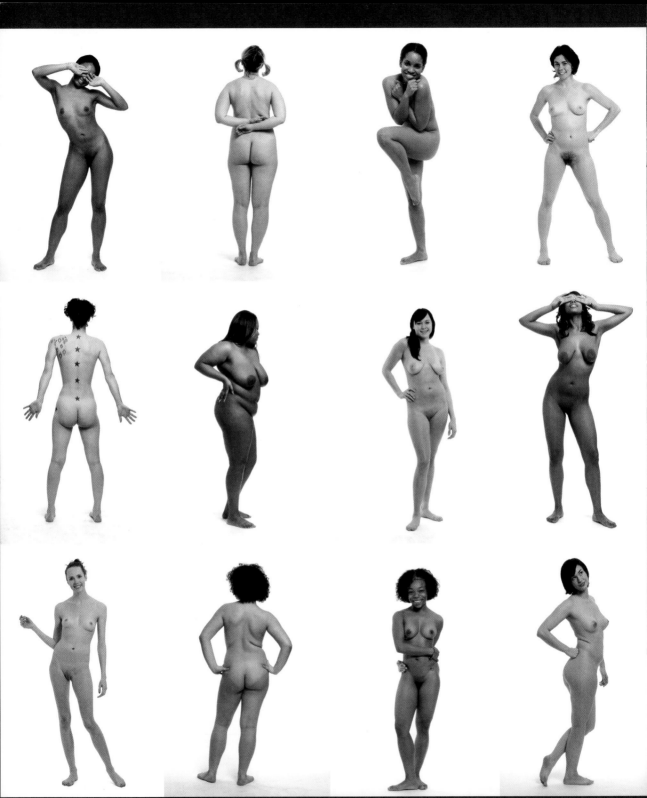

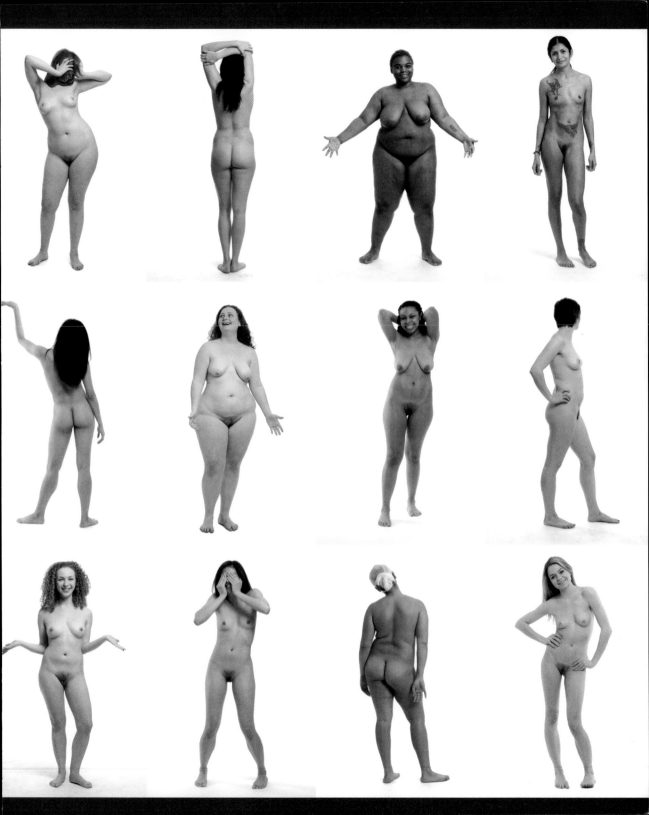

# RESOURCES

# ALL ABOUT DOCTORS
## (AND WHAT EACH KIND DOES)

Because this book is about body drama, I've written a lot about seeing the doctor. Everyone needs a relationship with a specific doctor who manages everyday health issues, makes referrals to medical specialists, and arranges admissions to the hospital when needed. Whenever you feel that something needs checking, your personal doctor will know your medical history best, and that's the person you should see first. Even if you're feeling well, see your doctor once a year for a routine physical checkup.

Don't have a doctor? Call (or have someone call) your insurance company to find out which doctors your policy pays for and how you can arrange care. Without insurance? Talk to your school counselor or nurse about your family's circumstances. Ask for help finding affordable—possibly free—healthcare services from places such as the Mount Sinai Adolescent Health Center in New York City that Dr. Angela Diaz runs.

## THAT'S CONFIDENTIAL! (OR IS IT?)

If your healthcare provider agrees to have a confidential relationship with you, this means that the symptoms, concerns, and issues you discuss, the records the provider keeps, and the treatment you are prescribed will not be disclosed to anyone without your consent. All persons over the age of eighteen are granted these rights, but confidentiality rights for minors vary across the country.

Many states have confidentiality laws that protect underage patients seeking drug and alcohol treatment, reproductive and sexual health care, and mental health services, but some states require parental/guardian notification of treatments or diagnoses given to persons under the age of eighteen. Other states make parental disclosure optional for certain issues (such as birth control), leaving the decision to share up to each healthcare provider on a case by case basis.

Your local doctor's office or clinic can tell you the confidentiality rules for minors in your state. If you are under eighteen and are worried about whether parental notification is mandatory, optional, or not allowed by your state law, call and ask before scheduling an appointment so you won't be caught by surprise.

If you live in a state that cannot guarantee or that denies confidentiality to minors, you may be able to convince your parent/guardian to grant permission for you to have a confidential relationship with your health care provider, enabling you to share with your parents only what you feel comfortable with while getting treatment. If confidentiality isn't possible, don't let embarrassment, fear, or shame keep you from getting checked out, even if your family's involvement seems scary. Your health must come first!

# HOW TO PREP FOR YOUR DOCTOR'S VISIT

**WRITE IT DOWN**

The more information your doctor has about you and your medical history, the better. It's easy to forget an important detail once you're in the doctor's office, so get yourself a notebook to keep track of contact information, questions, notes, medications, tests, your blood type, allergies—anything at all related to your health! Keeping track of everything might seem a bit silly at first but having a health history is the first step in taking charge of your own healthcare. This notebook will save you (and your doctor) a ton of time, and everyone will be very impressed!

*Before your next visit, write down the following:*

- All of your symptoms and concerns, how long they've existed and how severe they are. (Each bit of information will bring the doctor closer to understanding what the issue might be, so don't hold back!) Be as specific as you can. For example, "My stomach sometimes hurts" isn't nearly as useful to the doctor as "For the past two weeks, I've been getting jabs of intense pain in my stomach that last for an hour or two every other day. I notice it more after I eat. This past week it has happened more often than the week before."

- All serious illnesses or medical conditions, past or present, such as (but of course not limited to) mononucleosis, cancer, endometriosis, or IBS.

- A list of the medications you are currently taking and any that you are allergic to. This step is VERY important. In addition to setting off your own allergy, some medications can be dangerous if mixed.

- The questions you want your doctor to answer, whether related to the reason you're in there or any other more general health issues. Be clear in your own mind about your goals for the visit and what you want to walk away with. Don't be afraid and don't think that you're wasting the doctor's time. Take advantage of this opportunity to talk to a professional!

**MAKE SURE TO BRING**

- Photo ID
- Proof of insurance
- Parental permission form if needed (see previous page for information on confidentiality)
- Your notebook (with the information above) and an empty folder for prescriptions, medical records, test results, and other materials your doctor may give you
- Your calendar so you can schedule new appointments (if needed)
- Something to do or read while you wait

**TAKE BACK HOME**

- Confirmation of your next appointment (if necessary)
- Follow-up date for any test results
- Written prescriptions and specialist referrals
- Notes from your visit with any instructions from the doctor
- A sense of accomplishment for being proactive about your health!

# ALL TYPES OF DOCTORS

For all types of doctors, here's a cheat sheet full of information to help you remember who does what:

### PRIMARY CARE PHYSICIANS/GENERALISTS

**WHAT THEY DO**: Your personal doctor provides general medical care ranging from doing a routine checkup to prescribing allergy medicine to stitching up a wound. Types of primary care physicians (PCPs) and general practitioners (GPs) include (but are not limited to) family physicians, pediatricians, and internists. Sometimes, nurse practitioners or physician assistants handle most routine, daily health needs, consulting a doctor when more complex health issues arise.

**WHEN TO GO**: At least once a year for an annual checkup and whenever you feel ill or find something that worries you.

**WHAT TO EXPECT**: During your checkup, your healthcare provider will probably weigh you, take body measurements, and ask you about your lifestyle. Common topics include your eating habits, drug and alcohol use, sexual activity, and how much you exercise. Then, the provider will give you a painless physical exam, examining your breasts for lumps, checking your spine, and examining other body parts to make sure you're healthy. Blood and urine samples may be taken for a variety of tests, from cholesterol to sexually transmitted infections (STIs). Feel free to request a specific test if there's something worrying you.

If you are diagnosed with a condition that requires special treatment, you'll be referred to one of the following specialists:

### GYNECOLOGISTS/OBSTETRICIANS

**WHAT THEY DO**: These specialists keep the reproductive system in good working order. The gynecologist gives you pelvic exams and Pap tests and can help you with period problems, breast issues, and prescriptions for birth control. Some gynecologists provide care for pregnant women and deliver babies.

**WHEN TO GO**: Whenever you feel ill or find something down there that worries you, and at least once a year for an annual checkup once you become sexually active.

**WHAT TO EXPECT**: During your exam, your gynecologist will talk with you about the regularity of your period (know when the first day of your last one was), your diet and exercise habits, your sexual activity, and any specific issues you may have. You'll put on a medical gown that opens in the front for your breast exam. When it's time for your pelvic exam, your doctor will ask you to lie back, spread your legs, and scoot your bottom toward the end of the table. Your doctor may peek inside your vagina with a tool called a speculum and take a sample of cells from your cervix. The cells are checked by a pathologist in a procedure called a Pap test. The Pap test detects cervical cancers in their early stages. It saves thousands of lives annually. The speculum may feel cold and you may feel a quick pinch, but that should be all. Your doctor has performed this procedure thousands of times, and it will be over before you know it, so don't worry!

## PSYCHIATRISTS/PSYCHOLOGISTS/SOCIAL WORKERS/THERAPISTS/COUNSELORS

**WHAT THEY DO:** Psychiatrists are medical doctors; they can prescribe drugs that help with mental and emotional issues (see pages 224–229 for more information on these types of issues). Psychiatrists, psychologists, social workers, therapists, and counselors can all be very helpful when your problems seem too big to overcome. "Talk therapy" can help you understand, resolve, and work through your emotional issues. If you're feeling depressed or causing harm to yourself, have an eating disorder, or just need a professional shoulder to lean on, talk to your school counselor. If you need or want additional help, ask for a recommendation for a professional you can see outside of school.

**WHAT TO EXPECT:** A psychiatrist, psychologist, social worker, or counselor can't help you unless you share yourself, so expect a lot of questions and allow plenty of time to answer them. While "telling all" might seem overwhelming at first, know that your mental health professional needs to know you well. The more honest your talk, the more

beneficial the treatment will be. These are people who are trained to help.

## OPHTHALMOLOGISTS AND OPTOMETRISTS

**WHAT THEY DO:** They make sure your eyesight is clear, providing you with prescriptions for glasses and contacts if needed.

**WHEN TO GO:** At least once a year for an exam and perhaps more often if you have eyesight complications. Ask your school nurse if a vision specialist is coming to your school any time soon or if you can get a referral to an eye clinic near you. Many local organizations sponsor free eye exams from time to time.

**WHAT TO EXPECT:** Your ophthalmologist or optometrist will perform a variety of tests on you to determine whether your eyesight is a perfect 20/20, to prescribe glasses or contacts if needed, and to make sure you don't have an eye infection or other serious condition.

## DENTISTS

**WHAT THEY DO:** They treat and prevent problems with your gums, mouth, and teeth.

**WHEN TO GO:** Proper dental care requires a checkup every six months. Go right away if you have pain, excessive bleeding, or infection of the mouth, teeth, or gums.

**WHAT TO EXPECT:** In many dentists' offices, a dental assistant or dental hygienist removes plaque and tartar from the teeth, takes X-rays for the dentist to study, and gives teeth a professional polish to make them clean and bright. Then the dentist checks for cavities and repairs teeth if necessary. Both professionals will advise you on the best ways to care for your teeth.

## DERMATOLOGISTS

**WHAT THEY DO:** They take care of skin, nails, hair, and sweat glands.

**WHEN TO GO:** Your doctor may refer you if you have severe acne, heavy dandruff, excessive sweating, a mole or other body spot that requires further examination, or "tan-orexia."

**WHAT TO EXPECT:** The dermatologist will ask you about your habits, examine your skin, order laboratory tests to diagnose infections or skin cancer, and prescribe medicine if you need it.

## OTHER TYPES OF DOCTORS

Here are some other doctors you may encounter under certain circumstances:

- **ALLERGISTS** treat allergies to pollen, dust, and foods.

- **ANESTHESIOLOGISTS** put people to sleep and manage painkilling drugs and procedures, especially during surgery.

- **CARDIOLOGISTS** treat heart and circulatory system diseases.

- **ENDOCRINOLOGISTS** specialize in the body's hormonal system and disorders that arise when it's out of balance, such as thyroid disease and diabetes.

- **NEUROLOGISTS** treat disorders of the nervous system, such as multiple sclerosis or epilepsy.

- **ONCOLOGISTS** treat cancer.

- **ORTHOPEDISTS** treat bone and joint injuries (if you break a leg, for example).

- **OTOLARYNGOLOGISTS** treat problems with the ears, nose, and throat; they are also known as ENTs.

- **RADIOLOGISTS** interpret X-rays, CT scans, and MRI scans.

- **SURGEONS** repair, remove, or transplant body parts and organs.

- **UROLOGISTS** treat disorders of the urinary system.

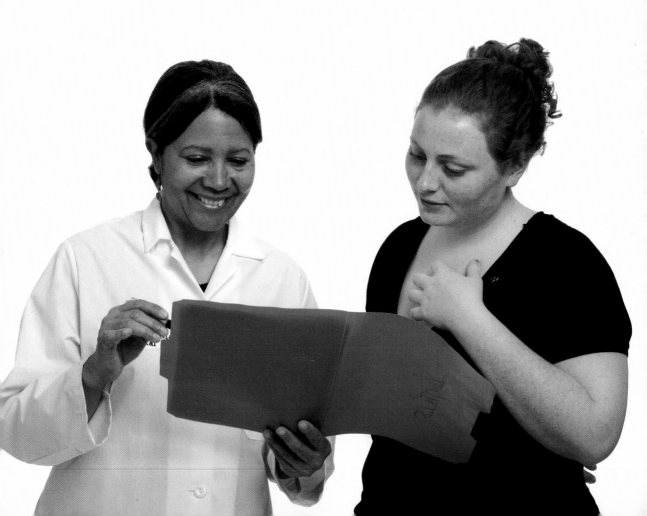

# ADDITIONAL RESOURCES

Besides this book and www.nancyredd.com, here are other fabulous resources, including phone numbers for free and confidential hotlines:

### ADD/ADHD
Attention Deficit Disorder
Association
www.add.org

### BODY PIERCING
Association of Professional
Piercers
www.safepiercing.org

### DRUGS AND ALCOHOL
Alcoholics Anonymous
www.aa.org

Cocaine Anonymous
www.ca.org

Marijuana Anonymous
www.marijuana-anonymous
.org

Narcotics Anonymous
www.na.org

Free Vibe
www.freevibe.com

National Drug Abuse Hotline
1-800-662-4357

Alcohol Abuse Hotline
1-800-ALCOHOL

The Cool Spot
www.thecoolspot.gov

### EATING DISORDERS
National Eating Disorders
Association
1-800-931-2237
www.edap.org

National Association of
Anorexia Nervosa
and Associated Disorders
1-847-831-3438
www.anad.org

Overeaters Anonymous
www.oa.org

### GENERAL ISSUES
Teen Central
www.teencentral.net/

### MENTAL HEALTH ISSUES
National Mental Health
Information Center
1-800-789-2647
mentalhealth.samhsa.gov

### SELF-INJURY
S.A.F.E. Alternatives
1-800-DONT CUT
www.selfinjury.com

### SEX, PREGNANCY, OR STIs
Planned Parenthood
1-800-230-PLAN
www.plannedparenthood.org

National Sexually Transmitted
Disease Hotline
1-800-227-8922

The Abstinence Clearinghouse
www.abstinence.net

American Social Health
Association
www.ashastd.org

### SEXUAL PREFERENCE
Gay, Lesbian, Bisexual, and
Transgender Youth Support
Line
1-800-850-8078

Safe Schools Coalition
www.safeschoolscoalition.org

### SKIN CARE
Skin Care Physicians
www.skincarephysicians.com

### SMOKING
American Cancer Society
1-877-YES-QUIT or
1-800-QUIT-NOW
www.cancer.org

## SUICIDE

National Suicide Hopeline
1-800-SUICIDE
www.hopeline.com

## TATTOOING

Alliance of Professional Tattooists
www.safe-tattoos.com

## VIOLENCE, SEXUAL HARASSMENT, OR ABUSE

Community United Against
Violence
1-415-333-HELP
www.cuav.org

Rape, Abuse, & Incest
National Network
1-800-656-HOPE
www.rainn.org

National Center for Victims
of Crime
1-800-FYI-CALL
www.ncvc.org/ncvc/Main
.aspx

National Domestic Violence
Hotline
1-800-799-SAFE
www.ndvh.org

National Teen Dating Abuse
Helpline
1-866-331-9474
loveisrespect.org

National Child Abuse Hotline
1-800-4-A-CHILD
www.childhelp.org

Founded in 1968, the
**Mount Sinai Adolescent
Health Center** has become
the largest freestanding
provider of outpatient
adolescent health services
in the U.S., and the only
one of its kind. The
center provides free and
comprehensive healthcare
each year to 10,000 urban
adolescents, ages ten
to twenty-one, in New
York City and beyond,
addressing their physical,
reproductive, emotional,
and mental health needs.
1-212-423-2900
www.mountsinai.org/
msh/msh_program.
jsp?url=clinical_services/
ahc.htm

Visit
www.NancyRedd.com
for even more resources
and information,
including

- a comprehensive list of
  state and local resources
  for mental and sexual
  health advice

- tips and support to quit
  smoking

- background information
  on the girls in the book

- more photos of real
  women's bodies

- a personal discharge
  calendar

- product reviews

- advice on how to wax and
  manicure at home

- recipes for masks and
  scrubs

- recipes and exercises to
  help you stay healthy

- and much, much more!

# NOTES

## SKIN

27  *"Skin is the largest organ"* Johns Hopkins Medicine, The Johns Hopkins Hospital, "Skin Disorders," http://www.hopkinshospital.org/health_info/Skin_Disorders/.

27  *"Thickest and thinnest skin"* Don R. Revis and Michael B. Seagle, "Skin, Anatomy," eMedicine from WebMD.com, February 17, 2006, http://www.emedicine.com/plastic/topic389.htm.

27  *"Skin layers"* Thomas J. Zuber, "Punch Biopsy of the Skin," *American Family Physician* 65 (March 15, 2002): 1155.

27  *"Skin cell loss"* "Human Skin," Discover.com, http://www.yucky.discovery.com/flash/body/pg000146.html.

29  *"Acne and infections"* U.S. National Library of Medicine and the National Institutes of Health, Medline Plus, "Acne," http://www.nlm.nih.gov/medlineplus/ency/article/000873.htm.

30  *"Men get worse acne than women"* National Women's Health Information Center, U.S. Department of Health and Human Services, Office on Women's Health, *Acne* (January 2006), http://www.4woman.gov/faq/acne.pdf.

36  *"Most warts disappear on their own"* WebMD, "Skin Conditions: Warts," http://www.webmd.com/content/article/117/112630.htm.

37  *"Herpes exposure"* Duane Swierczynski, "The STD You Already Have," *Men's Health* (2003), http://www.webmd.aol.com/genital-herpes/guide/herpes-std-you-already-have.

38  *"Hyperhidrosis"* Sid Kirchheimer, "Excessive Sweating: Embarrassing, Treatable: Nearly 8 Million Americans Affected, but Help Is Available," *WebMD Medical News*, July 29, 2004, http://www.webmd.com/content/article/91/101215.htm.

39  *"Hyperhidrosis treatment"* The Society of Thoracic Surgeons, "Patient Information: Hyperhidrosis," http://www.sts.org/sections/patientinformation/othersurgery/hyperhidrosis/.

41  *"Body odor"* "What Can I Do About My Strong Body Odor?" January 13, 2006, http://www.goaskalice.columbia.edu/3645.html.

41  *"Antiperspirants don't cause cancer"* National Cancer Institute, National Institutes of Health, "Antiperspirants/Deodorants and Breast Cancer: Questions and Answers," October 5, 2004, http://www.cancer.gov/cancertopics/factsheet/Risk/AP-Deo.

43  *"Effects of tanning"* American Academy of Dermatology, "The Darker Side of Tanning," U.S. Food and Drug Administration, Center for Devices and Radiological Health 1996, http://www.fda.gov/cdrh/consumer/tanning.html.

43  *"Teens and tanning"* Alan C. Geller, Graham Colditz, Susan Oliveria, Karen Emmons, Cynthia Jorgensen, Gideon N. Aweh, and A. Lindsay Frazier, "Use of Sunscreen, Sunburning Rates, and Tanning Bed Use Among More Than 10,000 U.S. Children and Adolescents," *Pediatrics* 109 (June 6, 2002): 1009-1014.

43  *"Melanoma"* The Melanoma Research Foundation, "Melanoma Fact Sheet," http://www.melanoma.org/upload/mrf_facts.pdf.

43  *"Sunburns increase risk for melanoma"* Julie Mitchell, "The Dark Side of the Sun: Sun Exposure and Agriculture," Oklahoma Agricultural Health, Promotion System, Department of Biosystems and Agricultural Engineering, Oklahoma State University, F-1712, http://www.cdc.gov/nasd/docs/d000701-d000800/d000769/d000769.pdf.

43  *"SPF and skin type"* American Academy of Dermatology, "Facts About Sunscreen," 2006, http://www.aad.org/aad/Newsroom/factsunscreen.htm.

44  *"Melanoma unrelated to sunbathing"* American Academy of Dermatology, "Melanoma in African Americans," May 3, 2004, http://www.aad.org/public/News/NewsReleases/Press+Release+Archives/Skin+Cancer+and+and+Sun+Safety/Melanoma_AfricanAmericans.htm.

46  *"Luxury tans"* "A Tan to Die For," BBC News, November 1, 2006, http://news.bbc.co.uk/2/hi/uk_news/magazine/6101740.stm.

50  *"Freckles"* Brynie, 1999, 98.

50  *"Epidermis"* Lars Norlén, "Reply: Letter to the Editor," *Journal of Investigative Dermatology* 118 (May 2002), 899–901.

51  *"Percent of women who complain of cellulite"* Anna Kuchment, "Health: When Dimples Go Bad," *Newsweek*, June 2005, http://www.findarticles.com/p/articles/mi_kmnew/is_200506/ai_n14760657.

52  *"Melanocytes"* Brynie, Faith, *101 Questions About Your Skin That Got Under Your Skin...Until Now* (Brookfield, CT: Twenty-First Century Books, 1999), 23.

52  *"Melanocyte activity in skin folds"* Julia Chance, "Skin Care by the Book," *Essence* (July 2004), http://www.findarticles.com/p/articles/mi_m1264/is_3_35/ai_n6094658.

53   *"Citric acid and skin cells"* Zoe Draelos and Joel Barkoff, "Hydroxy Acids," *Dialogues in Dermatology Commentaries* 52 (July 2003), http://www.aad.org/professionals/educationcme/AADCMEactivities/DialoguesDerm/DiDCommentJul2003.htm.

53   *"Vitiligo"* The National Institutes of Health, the National Institute of Arthritis and Musculoskeletal and Skin Diseases, "Questions and Answers about Vitiligo," October 2006, http://www.niams.nih.gov/hi/topics/vitiligo/vitiligo.htm.

53   *"Birthmarks"* Susan Peterson, "When a Birthmark Is Born: Researchers Find That Unique Marks Are Based on Genetics," *Harvard University Gazette*, March 27, 1997, http://www.hno.harvard.edu/gazette/1997/03.27/WhenaBirthmarki.html.

61   *"Piercing complications"* Lester B. Mayers, Daniel A. Judelson, Barry W. Moriarty, and Kenneth L. Rundell, "Prevalence of Body Art (Body Piercing and Tattooing) in University Undergraduates and Incidence of Medical Complications," *Mayo Clinic Proceedings* 77 (January 1, 2002) 29-34.

61   *"Piercing complications"* Donna I. Meltzer, "Complications of Body Piercing," *American Family Physician* 72 (November 15, 2005): 2029.

62   *"Suicide disease"* Roberto Gazzeri, Sandro Mercuri, and Marcelo Galarza, "Atypical Trigeminal Neuralgia Associated with Tongue Piercing," *Journal of the American Medical Association* 296 (October 18, 2006): 1840-1842.

63   *"Popularity of piercings"* Mayers et al, 2002.

63   *"Piercing healing times"* Meltzer, 2005.

## BOOBS

71   *"Humans develop breasts early"* Frances E. Mascia-Lees, "Are Women Evolutionary Sex Objects? Why Women Have Breasts" (December 5, 2002), http://www.nyu.edu/fas/ihpk/CultureMatters/Mascia-Lees.htm.

71   *"Breast changes during pregnancy"* M. Sara Rosenthal and Gillian Arsenault, "Breasts 101," WebMD.com, http://www.webmd.com/content/article/87/99611.htm?UID=%7BD3EF256F-F7B0-4AA3-AE55-7605BE6B7C94%7D.

81   *"Ashley Olsen taller than her twin"* Laurie Lynch, Whose News," USAWeekend.com (August 10, 2003), http://www.usaweekend.com/03_issues/030810/030810whosnews.html.

81   *"Difference in breast size"* C. W. Loughry, D. B. Sheffer, T. E. Price, R. L. Einsporn, R. G. Bartfai, W. M. Morek, and N. M. Meli, "Breast Volume Measurement of 598 Women Using Biostereometric Analysis," *Annals of Plastic Surgery* 22 (May 1989): 380.

82   *"Corset origination"* Britannica Concise, "Corset," http://concise.britannica.com/ebc/article-9361667/corset.

82   *"Mary Phelps Jacob"* Phelps Family History in America and Kindred Family Histories: Mary Phelps Jacob, Inventor of the Modern Brassiere," http://family.phelpsinc.com/bios/mary_phelps_jacob.htm.

82   *"Number of bras sold in America"* Anne Casselman, "The Physics of Bras: Overcoming Newton's Second Law with Better Bra Technology," *Discover* (November 22, 2005), http://www.discover.com/issues/nov-05/departments/physics-of-bras.

83   *"Special garments to show nipple jewelry"* Henry Ferguson, "Body Piercing," *British Medical Journal* 319 (December 18, 1999): 1627.

85   *"Polythelia"* J. M. Dixon and R. E. Mansel, "ABC of Breast Diseases: Congenital Problems and Aberrations of Normal Breast Development and Involution," *British Medical Journal* 309 (September 24, 1994): 797.

85   *"Polythelia by ethnicity"* Don R. Revis, "Breast Embryology," eMedicine from WebMD. http://www.emedicine.com/plastic/topic214.htm.

85   *"Links between polythelia and kidney disease"* J. R. Pellegrini and R. F. Wagner, "Polythelia and Associated Conditions," *American Family Physician* 28 (September 1983):129-132.

85   *"Links between polythelia and breast cancer"* Johns Hopkins Breast Center, "Scientists Identify Gene Involved in Breast Development" (October 2005), http://www.hopkinsbreastcenter.org/artemis/200510/14.html.

88   *"Breast weight"* Casselman, 2005.

91   *"Nipple icing"* Abigail Grenaway, "Star Slaves: I Couldn't Possibly..." *Sunday Mirror* (London), July 25, 2004, http://www.findarticles.com/p/articles/mi_qn4161/is_20040725/ai_n12900052.

92   *"The average woman owns about six bras"* The Genuine Article, Episode 107, "Undercover: La Perla Lingerie, Creed Perfume," http://www.fineliving.com/fine/genuine_article/episode/0,1663,FINE_1416_134,00.html.

95   *"Inverted nipples"* J. M. Alexander, A. M. Grant, and M. J. Campbell, "Randomised Controlled Trial of Breast Shells and Hoffman's Exercises for Inverted and Non-protractile Nipples," *British Medical Journal* 304 (April 18, 1992): 1030.

98   *"Breast soreness"* National Women's Health Information Center, U.S. Department of Health and Human Services, Office on Women's Health, "Body: Changes to Your Breasts," http://www.girlshealth.gov/body/changes_breasts.htm.

101  *"Nipple glands"* Rosenthal and Arsenault.

103  *"Nipple discharge"* U.S. National Library of Medicine and the National Institutes of Health, Medline Plus, "Nipple Discharge – Abnormal," http://www.nlm.nih.gov/medlineplus/ency/article/003154.htm.

104  "Breast lumps" St. Joseph Mercy Health System, "Noncancerous Breast Conditions," http://www.sjmercyhealth.org/body.cfm?id=276.

104  "Breast lumps" J. E. Devitt, T. To, and A. B. Miller, "Risk of Breast Cancer in Women with Breast Cysts," *Canadian Medical Association Journal* 147 (July 1992): 45-49.

105  "Fibrocystic breast disease" U.S. National Library of Medicine and the National Institutes of Health, Medline Plus, "Fibrocystic Breast Disease," http://www.nlm.nih.gov/medlineplus/ency/article/000912.htm.

105  "Baby boys are sometimes born with small breasts" Lucile Packard Children's Hospital at Stanford, "Newborn Appearance; Common Questions," http://www.lpch.org/HealthLibrary/ParentCareTopics/NewbornQuestions/NewbornAppearanceCommonQuestions.html.

## DOWN THERE

111  "Shock value of the vagina" Ibid, 5.

113  "Fewer than 50 percent of women have ever given themselves a simple self-exam" (The Association of Reproductive Health Professionals, *The Vagina Dialogues* (Harris Interactive, 2003), 10, http://www.arhp.org/files/vaginadialoguesresults.pdf.

113  "Ovarian eggs" "Genital Organs (Internal)," *The Merck Manuals Online Medical Library, Home Edition for Patients and Caregivers,* http://www.merck.com/mmhe/sec22/ch241/ch241c.html.

113  "Number of periods a woman will have in her lifetime" Lauri M. Aesoph, "Full Cycle: Taking the Mystery out of Menstruation," http://www.healthy.net/asp/templates/article.asp?PageType=Article&ID=375.

113  "Average number of tampons used in a lifetime" WebMD, "Menstrual Health: What You Ought to Know About Bleached Tampons," http://www.webmd.com/content/Article/85/98753.htm?pagenumber=3.

114  "Labiaplasty" Sandy Kobrin, "More Women Seek Vaginal Plastic Surgery," *Women's eNews*, November 14, 2004, http://www.womensenews.org/article.cfm/dyn/aid/2067/context/archive.

121  "Bartholin's duct cysts" Folashade Omole, Barbara J. Simmons, and Yolanda Hacker, "Management of Bartholin's Duct Cyst and Gland Abscess," *American* 68 (July 1, 2003), 135.

123  "HPV" Centers for Disease Control and Prevention, "Sexually Transmitted Diseases: Human Papillomavirus (HPV) Infection: Genital HPV Infection Fact Sheet," http://www.cdc.gov/STD/HPV/STDFact-HPV.htm.

123  "HPV vaccine" Centers for Disease Control and Prevention, "Sexually Transmitted Diseases: Human Papillomavirus (HPV) Infection: HPV Vaccine Questions and Answers," http://www.cdc.gov/std/hpv/STDFact-HPV-vaccine.htm#hpvvac1.

127  "Vaginal discharge" eMedicine from WebMD, "Excerpt from Vulvovaginitis," http://www.emedicine.com/emerg/byname/vulvovaginitis.htm.

129  "PID" National Institute of Allergy and Infectious Diseases, National Institutes of Health, "Pelvic Inflammatory Disease" (December 2005), http://www3.niaid.nih.gov/healthscience/healthtopics/pelvic/.

130  "STI contractions" Planned Parenthood, "Sexually Transmitted Infections," http://www.plannedparenthood.org/news-articles-press/politics-policy-issues/medical-sexual-health/Sexually-Transmitted-Infections.htm.

130  "STI contractions" Guttmacher Institute, "Facts on American Teens' Sexual and Reproductive Health" (September 2006), http://www.guttmacher.org/pubs/fb_ATSRH.html#ref23.

130  "Hepatitis B" Hepatitis B Foundation, "General Information: FAQ," http://www.hepb.org/patients/general_information.htm.

130  "Most common STIs" National Center for HIV, STD, and TB Prevention, Centers for Disease Control and Prevention, *Sexually Transmitted Disease Surveillance 2005* (November 2006), http://www.cdc.gov/std/stats/05pdf/Surv2005.pdf.

134  "Definition of heavy bleeding" A. L. Magos, "Management of Menorrhagia," *British Medical Journal* 300 (June 16, 1990), 1357.

134  "Definition of heavy bleeding" U.S. National Library of Medicine, National Institutes of Health, Medline Plus, "Menstrual Periods – Heavy, Prolonged, or Irregular," http://www.nlm.nih.gov/medlineplus/ency/article/003263.htm.

135  "TSS" Dixie Farley, "On the Teen Scene: TSS: Reducing the Risk," *FDA Consumer* (October 1991), http://www.fda.gov/bbs/topics/consumer/con00116.html.

138  "Cramps" Association of Reproductive Health Professionals, "2005 Menstruation Survey," http://www.arhp.org/2005MenstruationSurvey/fullreport.cfm.

138  "Purpose of cramps" Marian Segal, "On the Teen Scene: A Balanced Look at the Menstrual Cycle," *FDA Consumer* (December 1993), http://www.fda.gov/fdac/reprints/ots_mens.html.

141  "PMS" U.S. Department of Health and Human Services, Office on Women's Health, "Premenstrual Syndrome," http://www.4women.gov/faq/pms.pdf.

141  "85 percent PMS" U.S. Department of Health and Human Services, Office on Women's Health, "Premenstrual Syndrome," http://www.4women.gov/faq/pms.pdf.

141  "Diet and supplements" Ibid.

143  "Sexual activity before marriage" Lawrence B. Finer, "Trends in Premarital Sex in the United States, 1954–2003," *Public Health Reports* 122 (January–February 2007), 73.

144  *"Contraception"* All estimates for contraceptive failure rates are taken from the Planned Parenthood Web site at www .plannedparenthood.org.

144  *"Teenage pregnancy"* The Guttmacher Institute, *U.S. Teenage Pregnancy Statistics National and State Trends and Trends by Race and Ethnicity* (New York: The Guttmacher Institute, 2006), http://www.teenpregnancy.org/resources/data/pdf/pregrate_Oct2006.pdf.

147  *"UTIs"* National Kidney and Urologic Diseases Information Clearinghouse, "Urinary Tract Infections in Adults," http://kidney.niddk.nih.gov/kudiseases/pubs/utiadult/.

149  *"Fiber"* Ruth Papazian, "Bulking Up Fiber's Healthful Reputation: More Benefits of 'Roughage' Are Discovered," *FDA Consumer* (July-August 1997), http://www.fda.gov/fdac/features/1997/597_fiber.html.

149  *"Bowel movements during menstruation"* Amanda L. P Vlitos and G. Jill Davies, "Bowel Function, Food Intake and the Menstrual Cycle," Nutrition Research Reviews 9 (January 1996), 112.

150  *"Celiac Disease"* Celiac Disease Foundation, "Celiac Disease," http://www.celiac.org/downloads/CDF_05_Brochure.pdf.

150  *"IBS"* National Digestive Diseases Information Clearinghouse, "Irritable Bowel Syndrome," http://digestive.niddk.nih.gov/ddiseases/pubs/ibs/.

150  *"IBD"* Amber J. Tresca, "Arthritis and IBD," http://ibdcrohns.about.com/cs/relatedconditions/a/arthritisibd.htm; National Institutes of Health, Osteoporosis and Related Bone Diseases, National Resource Center, "What People with Inflammatory Bowel Disease Need to Know About Osteoporosis," November 2006, http://www.niams .nih.gov/bone/hi/bowel/ibd.htm.

151  *"Half have hemorrhoids"* U.S. National Library of Medicine and the National Institutes of Health, Medline Plus, "Hemorrhoids," http://www.nlm.nih.gov/medlineplus/hemorrhoids.html.

154  *"Gas fourteen times daily"* National Institute of Diabetes and Digestive and Kidney Diseases, National Institutes of Health., "Gas in the Digestive Tract," http://digestive.niddk .nih.gov/ddiseases/pubs/gas/index.htm

## HAIR

159  *"Number of scalp hairs"* Brynie, Faith, *101 Questions About Your Skin That Got Under Your Skin...Until Now* (Brookfield, CT: Twenty-First Century Books, 1999), 40.

159  *"Number of scalp hairs by hair color"* Ibid.

159  *"Dental imprints"* D. K. Whittaker, "Bite Marks—The Criminal's Calling Cards," *British Dental Journal* 196 (February 28, 2004): 237.

162  *"'Pubic' typo"* Associated Press, "'Pubic' Typo Will Cost Michigan County $40,000," October 10, 2006, http://abclocal.go.com/ktrk/story?section=bizarre&id=4647225.

163  *"Merkin"* "The History of the Merkin," http://www .merkinworld.com/history_01.htm.

165  *"Best time of day to shave"* National Women's Health Resource Center, "Teen Health," http://www .healthywomen.org/healthtopics/teenhealth.

171  *"Body hair"* "Molecular Signatures of the Developing Hair Follicle," *PLoS Biology* 3 (November 2005):e3666, http://www.pubmedcentral.nih.gov/articlerender .fcgi?artid=1216329.

171  *"Types of body hair"* Howard P. Baden, "Structure and Function of Hair Follicles," http://www.aad .org/professionals/Residents/MedStudCoreCurr/DCHairFollicles.htm.

176  *"HPV found on the underwear of infected invidivuals"* New York State Department of Health, "Questions and Answers About Human Papillomavirus (HPV) Vaccine," http://www.health.state.ny.us/prevention/immunization/human_papillomavirus/.

177  *"Infections from salons"* Ilene Lelchuk and Elizabeth Fernandez, "Dirty Foot Spas a Danger in Pedicures," *San Francisco Chronicle*, August 10, 2006, http://sfgate.com/cgi-bin/article.cgi?f=/c/a/2006/08/10/PEDICURE.TMP.

181  *"Alopecia"* National Institute of Arthritis and Musculoskeletal and Skin Diseases (NIAMS), National Institutes of Health, *Questions and Answers About Alopecia Areata*, NIH Publication No. 03-5143 (February 2003), http://www.niams.nih.gov/hi/topics/alopecia/alopecia .htm.

181  *"Hair loss"* U.S. National Library of Medicine and the National Institutes of Health, Medline Plus, "Hair Loss," http://www.nlm.nih.gov/medlineplus/ency/article/003246.htm.

182  *"Scalp shedding"* T. Hingley, "OTC Options: Controlling Dandruff," *FDA Consumer* (October 1994), http://www .fda.gov/bbs/topics/CONSUMER/CON0290d.html.

182  *"Dandruff"* Mayo Clinic, "Dandruff," http://www .mayoclinic.com/health/dandruff/DS00456.

185  *"Nail biting"* "Nail Biting," *Gale Encyclopedia of Childhood and Adolescence*, Gale Research, 1998, http://findarticles.com/p/articles/mi_g2602/is_0003/ai_2602000393.

185  *"Trichotillomania"* Trichotillomania Learning Center, "About Trichotillomania," http://www.trich.org/about_trich/.

185  *"Nail color and social class in ancient China"* "Nail Polish Trends," CBS News: The Early Show, August 4, 2003, http://www.cbsnews.com/stories/2003/08/04/earlyshow/living/beauty/main566623.shtml.

186  *"Fingernails grow faster than toenails"* Fernando Barbosa, Jr, José Eduardo Tanus-Santos, Raquel Fernanda Gerlach, and Patrick J. Parsons, "A Critical Review of Biomarkers Used for Monitoring Human Exposure to Lead: Advantages, Limitations, and Future Needs," *Environmental Health Perspectives* 113 (December 2005): 1669.

186  *"Nail color and health"* Sherry Rauh, "What Your Nails Say About Your Health," WebMD.com, http://www.webmd.com/content/article/101/106448.htm?z=4209_00000_5022_pe_02.

187  *"Onychomycosis"* "Onychomycosis," *The Merck Manuals Online Medical Library, The Merck Manual for Healthcare Professionals,* http://www.merck.com/mmpe/sec10/ch125/ch125c.html.

189  *"Tooth enamel"* U.S. National Library of Medicine, "Genetics Home Reference: Your Guide to Understanding Genetic Conditions: Enamel," March 9, 2007, http://ghr.nlm.nih.gov/ghr/glossary/enamel.

190  *"Underage tooth whitening"* Massachusetts Dental Society, "When It Comes to Whitening, Age Should Come Before Beauty," to http://www.massdental.org/uploadedFiles/5_Publications/Word_of_Mouth/Summer-Fall_2006/WOM_whitening.pdf.

190  *"Saliva"* Discovery Education, "Human Biology: Digest This," Discoveryschool.com, http://school.discovery.com/studystarters/facts/humanbio_digestthis.html.

190  *"Braces"* Linda Bren, "Straight Talk on Braces," *FDA Consumer* (January-February 2005), http://www.fda.gov/fdac/features/2005/105_braces.html.

193  *"Teens who start smoking"* American Cancer Society, *No Ifs, Ands, or Butts: A Guide to Tobacco Use Prevention,* http://www.cancer.org/downloads/COM/JrHSGASOCurriculum.pdf.

193  *"One in five teens are currently regular smokers"* National Center for Chronic Disease Prevention and Health Promotion, Tobacco Information and Prevention Source (TIPS), "Teens and Tobacco: Facts Not Fiction," http://www.worthit.org/facts/teenstobacco.asp.

## SHAPE

199  *"Fat cell storage"* Royal Society of Chemistry, "Fat of the Land," *Chemistry World,* December 2006, http://www.rsc.org/chemistryworld/Issues/2006/December/FatOfLand.asp.

199  *"Necessity of body fat for menstruation"* P. Klentrou and M. Plyley, "Onset of Puberty, Menstrual Frequency, and Body Fat in Elite Rhythmic Gymnasts Compared with Normal Controls," *British Journal of Sports Medicine* 37 (December 2003): 490-494.

202  *"BMI"* Emma Seifret Weigley, "Adolphe Quetelet: Pioneer Anthropometrist - 1796-1874," *Nutrition Today* (April, 1989).

206  *"Cost of being overweight"* Rachel N. Close and Dale A. Schoeller, "The Financial Reality of Overeating," *Journal of the American College of Nutrition* 25 (June 2006): 203-209.

206  *"Emotional aspect of weight"* National Center for Health Statistics, Centers for Disease Control, "Obesity Still a Major Problem," April 14, 2006, http://www.cdc.gov/nchs/pressroom/06facts/obesity03_04.htm.

206  *"Emotional aspect of weight"* Girl Scouts of the USA, "Girls Aspire to be 'Normal Healthy,' According to New Girl Scout Research Institute Study," January 25, 2006, http://www.girlscouts.org/news/news_releases/2006/healthy_living.asp.

206  *"60 percent of adult Americans are overweight"* National Institutes of Health, "Vast Majority of Adults at Risk of Becoming Overweight or Obese," *NIH News,* October 3, 2005, http://www.nih.gov/news/pr/oct2005/nhlbi-03.htm.

211  *"Food allergies"* National Institute of Allergy and Infectious Diseases, National Institutes of Health, *Food Allergy: An Overview* (NIH: July 2004), 6, http://www.niaid.nih.gov/publications/pdf/foodallergy.pdf.

212  *"Portion size"* Lisa R. Young and Marion Nestle, "The Contribution of Expanding Portion Sizes to the U.S. Obesity Epidemic," American Journal of Public Health 92 (February 2002): 246–249.

213  *"Daily Reference Value"* Paula Kurtzweil, " 'Daily Values' Encourage Healthy Diet," http://www.fda.gov/FDAC/special/foodlabel/dvs.html.

215  *"Metabolism"* U.S. National Library of Medicine and the National Institutes of Health, Medline Plus, "Physical Activity," http://www.nlm.nih.gov/medlineplus/ency/article/001941.htm.

220  *"Underweight individuals"* Charlotte A. Schoenborn, Patricia F. Adams, and Patricia M. Barnes, "Body Weight Status of Adults: United States, 1997–98," *CDC, Advance Data from Vital and Health Statistics* 330 (September 6, 2002).

220  *"Average height and weight"* National Center for Health Statistics, FastStats A-Z, http://www.cdc.gov/nchs/fastats/bodymeas.htm.

220  *"Models' height and weight"* Nanci Hellmich, "Do Thin Models Warp Girls' Body Image?" *USA Today* (September 26, 2006), http://www.usatoday.com/news/health/2006-09-25-thin-models_x.htm.

221  *"Unhealthy methods of weight control"* D. Neumark-Sztainer, P. Hannan, M. Story, C. Perry. "Weight-Control Behaviors among Adolescent Girls and Boys: Implications for Dietary Intake," *Journal of the American Dietetic Association* 104 (June 2004): 913-920.

221  *"Anorexia"* Dixie Farley, "On the Teen Scene: Eating Disorders Require Medical Attention," *FDA Consumer,* March 1992, http://www.fda.gov/fdac/reprints/eatdis.html.

221  *"Death and eating disorders"* U.S. National Library of Medicine and the National Institutes of Health: Medline Plus, "Anorexia Nervosa," http://www.nlm.nih.gov/medlineplus/ency/article/000362.htm.

221  *"Bulimia"* Farley, 1992.

222  *"Binge eating disorder"* J. F. Kinzl, C. Traweger, E. Trefalt, B. Mangweth, and W. Biebl, "Binge Eating Disorder in Females: A Population-based Investigation. *International Journal of Eating Disorders* 25 (April 1999): 287-292.

222  *"Compulsive overeating"* Food and Nutrition Information Center, National Agricultural Library, USDA, "Eating Disorders: a Food and Nutrition Resource List for Consumers," (July 2001) http://www.nal.usda.gov/fnic/pubs/bibs/gen/eatingdis.htm#Binge.

222 *"10 million women have eating disorders"* National Eating Disorders Association, "Statistics: Eating Disorders and their Precursors," http://www.nationaleatingdisorders.org:80/p.asp?WebPage_ID=286&Profile_ID=41138.

223 *"Effects of teenage dieting on adult weight"* D. Neumark-Sztainer, M. Wall, J. Guo, M. Story, J. Haines, and M. Eisenberg. "Obesity, Disordered Eating, and Eating Disorders in a Longitudinal Study of Adolescents: How Do Dieters Fare 5 Years Later?" *Journal of the American Dietetic Association* 106 (April 2006): 559-568.

223 *"Side effects of weight-loss supplements"* Janet Heinrich, "Dietary Supplements for Weight Less: Limited Federal Oversight Has Focused More on Marketing than on Safety," Testimony Before the Subcommittee on Oversight of Government Management, Restructuring, and the District of Columbia, Committee on Governmental Affairs, U.S. Senate (July 31, 2002), http://www.gao.gov/new.items/d02985t.pdf.

223 *"Supplements aren't regulated"* Federal Trade Commission, "Weight Loss Advertising: An Analysis of Current Trends," (September 2002), http://www.ftc.gov/bcp/reports/weightloss.pdf.

223 *"Health problems from supplements"* "Supplements Associated with Illnesses and Injuries," *FDA Consumer* (September - October 1998), http://www.cfsan.fda.gov/~dms/fdsuppch.html

223 *"Billion dollar industry"* Jane E. Brody, "Weight-Loss Drugs: Hoopla and Hype," *New York Times* ( April 24, 2007) "http://www.nytimes.com/2007/04/24/health/24brod.html?ex=1183867200&en=66b5ab4ad1553ec5&ei=5070.

224 *"Depression"* Shashi K. Bhatia and Subhash C. Bhatia, "Childhood and Adolescent Depression," *American Family Physician* 75 (January 1, 2007), 73.

224 *"20 percent experience depression"* National Alliance on Mental Illness, "Depression in Children and Adolescents,"http://www.nami.org/Template.cfm?Section=By_Illness&template=/ContentManagement/ContentDisplay.cfm&ContentID=17623.

225 *"Reasons for depression"* U.S. National Library of Medicine and the National Institutes of Health, Medline Plus, "Adolescent Depression," http://www.nlm.nih.gov/medlineplus/ency/article/001518.htm.

226 *"Types of depression"* National Institute of Mental Health, National Institutes of Health, "Depression," http://www.nimh.nih.gov/publicat/depression.cfm

228 *"Methods of self-injury"* "Hurting Yourself," http://www.4girls.gov/mind/help.injury.htm.

229 *"Self harm statistics"* Keith Hawton and Emma Evans, "Deliberate Self Harm in Adolescents: Self Report Survey in Schools in England," *British Medical Journal* 325 (November 23, 2002): 1207–1211.

229 *"Growth of self harm"* Amanda Purington and Janis Whitlock, "Self-Injury Fact Sheet," ACT for Youth Upstate Center of Excellence, *Research Facts and Findings*, August 2004, http://www.actforyouth.net/documents/fACTS_Aug04.pdf.

229 *"Rate of female drug and alcohol abuse"* Office of National Drug Control Policy, Executive Office of the President, *Girls and Drugs: A New Analysis: Recent Trends, Risk Factors and Consequences,* February 9, 2006, http://www.mediacampaign.org/pdf/girls_and_drugs.pdf.

230 *"Teenage physical assault statistics"* The National Center for Victims of Crime, "Teen Victims," http://www.ncvc.org/ncvc/main.aspx?dbName=DocumentViewer&DocumentID=38721.

230 *"Ages 12-19 largest percentage of rape victims"* Ibid.

230 *"Rape every eight minutes"* Rape, Abuse & Incest National Network (RAINN), "Every Two and a Half Minutes," http://www.rainn.org/statistics/minutes.html.

230 *"Unreported sexual assault"* Rape, Abuse & Incest National Network (RAINN), "Statistics: Key Facts," http://www.rainn.org/statistics/index.html.

230 *"Types of sexual assault"* "Sexual Assault" www.4woman.gov/faq/sexualassault.htm.

230 *"Teenage sexual assault statistics"* The National Center for Victims of Crime, "Teen Victims," http://www.ncvc.org/ncvc/main.aspx?dbName=DocumentViewer&DocumentID=38721.

233 *"BDD"* Katharine A. Phillips, "Body Dysmorphic Disorder: Recognizing and Treating Imagined Ugliness," *World Psychiatry* 3 (February 2004): 12–17.

237 *"Number of teenage cosmetic surgeries"* R. Merrel Olesen and Marie B. V. Olesen, *Cosmetic Surgery for Dummies* (New York: Wiley, 2005), 14-15.

238 *"Liposuction fatalities"* F. M. Grazer and R. H. de Jong, "Fatal Outcomes from Liposuction: Census Survey of Cosmetic Surgeons," *Plastic and Reconstructive Surgery* 105 (January 2000): 436-446.

*"Pronunciations"* All pronunciations are taken from the Dictionary.com Web site. Dictionary.com *Unabridged (v 1.1)*. Random House, Inc. http://dictionary.reference.com.

# ACKNOWLEDGMENTS

Tremendous thanks to my mommy, Amanda, my brother Sammy, and my main squeeze, Rupak, for supporting me through thick and thin (and everything between); to the fabulously talented Caroline Herter of Herter Studio for "getting it," making it better, and also for making it happen (no one else could have!); to Debbie Berne of Herter Studio for her incredible design and for keeping us all sane and on track; to Kelly Kline for her courage, camaraderie, and awesome photographs; and to Faith Brynie for her eagle-eye and patience!

To Dr. Angela Diaz, for her extraordinary expertise, inspiration, encouragement, and generosity . . . it has been such an honor for me to work with you; to her colleagues at Mt. Sinai, Nora Helfgott and John Steever, for their valuable medical advice; and to Dr. Virgie Ellington for being there in the beginning.

To the incredibly open-minded and supportive Hilary Terrell and Bill Shinker of Gotham for publishing me and letting me keep the vaginas, and to Jessica Sindler for being a fabulous pinch hitter!

To Don Floyd and Lynn Luckow of 4-H for generously introducing me to Herter Studio; to my mentor, Lynn Berry, and the 4-H Program for giving me the opportunity to achieve as a teen; to my high school English teacher, Mrs. Gail Oakes, for encouraging my creativity; and to the Harvard Women's Studies Department (now Studies of Women, Gender, and Sexuality) for challenging and supporting me through everything.

Of course, to all the amazing young women who dared to bare for this great cause (and to www.craigslist.org, without which we never would have found one another!); and last but not least, a big thanks to all the girls, young and old, who I've encountered over the years, and who candidly shared their issues with me, helping me to realize that I wasn't the only one with body drama and that this book really needed to happen.

# PHOTOGRAPHY CREDITS

**Persons whose photos appear in this book are over the age of eighteen.**

# INDEX

**Note:** Page numbers in *italics* refer to illustrations.

## A

abdominal crunches, 217
abstinence, sexual, 130
acne
    and birth control pills, 140
    body acne, 34–35
    facial acne, 28–33
    and melanocytes, 52
    scarring from, 35
    and smoking, 193
airbrushed photos, *240–43*
alcohol abuse, 229, 256
alopecia, 181
American Cancer Society, 193
anal sex, 151
anorexia, 221
antiperspirants, 38, 39, 41, 42
anus, 117, 151
anxiety disorders, 39
apocrine glands, 41
appearance, obsession with,
    232–34
aspirin, 32–33
assaults, 230–31
author stories, 17–21, 51,
    120, 125, 175, 208, 227,
    235

## B

bacne, 34, *35*
bacterial vaginosis (BV), 124,
    125, 128
Bartholin's duct cysts, *121*

basal metabolic rate (BMR),
    215
bathroom, going to. *See*
    defecation; urinary tract
    infections (UTI)
benzoyl peroxide, 29
binge eating, 222
birth control pills, 73, 140.
    *See also* contraception
birthmarks, 53
blackheads, *31*
bloating, 140
body acne, 34–35
body dysmorphic disorder,
    233
body image, 204
body mass index (BMI), 202
body odor, 40–42
boobs. *See* breasts
bowel movements. *See* defeca-
    tion
braces, 190
bras
    bra fit, *92*, 92–93, 97
    and breast discomfort, 99
    and cleavage, 85, 88, *88*
    cup sizes, 74, 92, 97
    and different-sized breasts,
        81, 82
    history of, 82
    for large-breasted women,
        78
    and nipple erections, 91
    padding in, 74
    wearing no bra, 93
breasts, 69–107
    about, 70–71

breast cancer, 103, 104–5,
    106–7
breast exams, 105, *106–7*
breast ironing, 89
breast reduction surgery,
    78–79, *79*
bumps on, 101
cleavage, 84–85, *88*, 88
components of, 71
discomfort, 77–78, 98–99
emoticons, 100
itching of, 98–99
lumps in, 98, 104–5
nicknames, 75
sagging breasts, 86–88
size of, 71, 72–74, 76–79,
    80–83, 88
*See also* bras; nipples
breath, 191–92, 193
bulimia, 221
bumps or lumps
    on anus, 151
    on breasts, 98, 101, 104–5
    on vulva, 120, 121–22
buttne, 34, *35*

## C

calluses, *36*, 36
Cameroon, Africa, 89
cancer
    and antiperspirants, 41
    breast cancer, 103, 104–5,
        106–7
    and human papilloma virus,
        123, 143
    skin cancer, 43–45, *44*, *45*
    and smoking, 193

candidiasis, 124, 128
carrots, 58
celiac disease, 150
cellulite, 51, 56–58
cervix, 117
chlamydia, 128, 130, 131
citric acid, 53, 59
cleavage, 84–85, 88, *88*
clitoris, 111, 114, 116, 117,
    *117*
clothing
    and acne, 34–35
    and breast discomfort, 99
    and breast size, 77
    and cellulite, 58
    and darker skin colors, 53
    and nipple erections, 91
    and odors, 41, 125
    panties, 137, 151, 153–54,
        *155*
    sizes, 197, 203
    and sweat, 38, 39
    and yeast infections, 128
coffee grounds body scrub, 59
cold sores, 37
compulsive overeating, 222
condoms, 130, 143, 145
constipation, 140, 148, 149,
    151
contraception
    birth control pills, 73, 140
    and breast size, 73
    condoms, 130, 143, 145
    emergency contraception,
        145
    and tampons, 135
    types of, 144–45

corns, *36*, 36
cosmetic surgery, 79, 115,
    236–41
cutting. *See* self injury
crabs, 130, 168–69, *169*
cramps, 138–39, 140
Crohn's disease, 150
crunches, *217*
cysts, *31*, 98, 99, 105, *121*

**D**

dandruff, 182–83
defecation
    bathroom deodorizers, 154
    common problems, 150
    constipation, 140, 148, 149,
        151
    diarrhea, 148, 149, 151
    discomfort during, 149, 150,
        151
    frequency of, 148–49
    and hygiene, 153–54
    and skidmarks, 153–54
deodorants, 38, 41, 42
depilatories, 173
depression, 224–27
diarrhea, 148, 149, 151
Diaz, Angela, 13–15, 20
dieting, 220. *See also* nutrition
diet pills, 223
discharge, 99, 102–3, 124,
    126–29
doctors, 30, 39, 250–51,
    252–54, 255
douching, 129

"down there," 110–13, 116–17.
    *See also* defecation; men-
    struation; vagina; vulva
drinking. *See* alcohol abuse
drug use, 159, 229, 256
dry skin, 54–55
dysmenorrhea, 138

**E**

eating disorders, 218–23, 256
eggs, 113
electrolysis, 175
emoticons, 100, 152
emotional health
    anxiety disorders, 39
    depression, 224–27
    eating disorders, 218–23,
        256
    and professional help, 227,
        231
    self-injury, 228–29
endometriosis, 139
Ensler, Eve, 124
exercise
    and acne, 29, 30, 34–35
    and bloating, 140
    and cellulite, 58
    and menstruation, 141
    and metabolism, 215, 216
    and posture, 78, *78*
    and sports bras, 93
    and stress, 30
    and weight loss, 207,
        210–11
exfoliation, 29, 53, 59
eyebrow tweezing, 172, *172*

# INDEX

nicknames, 133
number of cycles, 113
and panty stains, 137
premenstrual syndrome (PMS), 141
products for, 113, 135, 142
and toxic shock syndrome, 135
and weight, 199
metabolism, 214–16, 220
moisturizers, 50, 53, 55, 58
moles, *36, 36,* 44
mons, 111
Mount Sinai Adolescent Health Center, 13, 20, 257
mouth, 62–63, 188–90, 191–92, 193
muffin tops, 203

## N

nails, 177, 184–86, 187
Nancy Redd. *See* author stories
National Center for Victims of Crime, 230
National Family Planning & Reproductive Health Association, 132
nicknames, 75, 119, 133
nipples
 bumps around, 101
 development of, 73
 discharge from, 99, 102–3
 erect nipples, 90–91
 hair on, 91
 inverted nipples, 94–96
 piercings, 63, 83, 96
 third nipples, 85

*See also* breasts
nodules, *31*
nutrition
 and bad breath, 191–92
 and bloating, 140
 and breast development, 74
 and breast lumps, 105
 and dieting, 220
 and eating disorders, 218–23, 256
 and food sensitivities, 211
 and hair, 179
 and menstruation, 141, 142
 and metabolism, 215–16
 nutrition labels, 213
 and odors, 38, 41
 and portion control, 212
 and super-sizing meals, 199
 and urine, 147
 and weight, 207, 211–12, 213

## O

obesity, 202
odors, 38, 40–42, 124–25, 128
oily skin, 30
onychomycosis, 187
onychophagia, 184–86
oral sex, 37, 130
ovaries, 113
overeating. *See* cumpulsive overeating

## P

panties, 137, 151, 153–54, *155*
papules, *31*
peeing, pain while, 146–47

pelvic inflammatory disease (PID), 124, 129
periods. *See* menstruation
pheromones, 161
photography, *240–43*
physical assault, 230
piercings, 60–65, 83, 96, 256
pimples. *See* acne
Planned Parenthood, 132
plastic surgery. *See* cosmetic surgery
polythelia, 85
poo. *See* defecation
pornography, 112, 114
portion control, 212
posture, 77, 78–79
pregnancy, 142, 143, 256
premenstrual syndrome (PMS), 141
ptosis, 86–88
pubic hair, 114, 115, *117,* 117, 160–63
pubic lice, 131
pulling hair out (trichotillomania), 184–86
pustules, *31*

## Q

queefing, 127

## R

rape, 230–31, 257
razor burn, 164–167
resources, 132, 256–57
role models, 14
rough skin, 54–55

# INDEX

## S

salicylic acid, 29
salons, 176–77
scales, 235
scams, 51
scars, 35
scrubs, 59
sebaceous glands, 28
seborrheic dermatitis, 183
sebum, 28, 34
secondary amenorrhea, 142
secretions, vaginal, 124,
   126–29
self-injury, 228–29
sex
   and abstinence, 130
   being sexually active, 37,
      143
   birth control (*see*
      contraception)
   and breasts, 88, 91
   and pregnancy, 142, 143,
      256
   resources, 132, 256
   *See also* sexually transmitted
      infections (STIs)
sexual abuse. *See* sexual assualt
sexual assault, 230–31, 257
sexually transmitted infections
   (STIs)
   about, 130–31
   chlamydia, 128, 130, 131
   and condoms, 130, 143
   gonorrhea, 128, 130, 131
   hepatitis, 130
   herpes, 37, *122*, 130

HIV, 130
human papilloma virus, 36,
   *122*, 123, 130, 143
lice, 130, 168–69, *169*
and pelvic inflammatory
   disease, 129
and rape, 231
resources, 132, 256
syphilis, 130
testing for, 131, 143
trichomoniasis, 128, 130
warts, *122*, 123, 143
sexual preference, 256
shame, 111, 112
shape, 194–244
   about, 196–99
   and body image, 204
   and body mass index (BMI),
      202
   and cosmetic surgery, 115,
      236–39
   and crunches, *217*
   and feeling fat, 200–203
   and managing fitness,
      209–13
   and metabolism, 214–16,
      220
   reactions to, 208
   *See also* nutrition; weight
shaving, 52, 115, 165, 166–67
skid marks in panties, 153–54
skin, 26–67
   about, 26–27
   acne, 28–33, 34–35, 52,
      140, 193
   calluses and corns, 36, *36*
   cellulite, 51, 56–58

cold sores, 37
darker skin, 52–53
dry, rough skin, 54–55
and facials, 32–33, 59
moles, 36, *36*, 44
odors, 38, 40–42
oily skin, 30
and piercings, 60–65, 83,
   96, 256
resources, 256
skin cancer, 43–45, *44*, *45*
and skin care products, 59
and smoking, 55, 193
stretch marks, 48–51, 58
sweat, 34–35, 38–39, 41
and tanning, 43–47, 55, 58
and tattoos, 66–67, 257
warts, 36, *36*
sleep, 141
smoking
   about, 193
   and bad breath, 192
   and birth control pills, 140
   resources, 257
   and skin, 55, 193
   and teeth color, 190
spermicide, 144. *See also* contraception
stress
   and acne, 28, 30
   and dandruff, 183
   and depression, 225
   and food, 222
   and menstruation, 141, 142
   and sweat, 38
stretch marks, 48–51, 58
substance abuse. *See* drug use

## NANCY REDD

Two weeks after graduating from Harvard with an honors degree in women's studies, author Nancy Redd won the title of Miss Virginia, going on to make the top ten and winning the swimsuit competition at Miss America 2004. Nancy has been named one of *Glamour* magazine's Top Ten College Women, L'OREAL's Beauty of Giving Young Woman of the Year, and one of *Harvard* magazine's Top Six Seniors. Nancy once won $250,000 on *Who Wants to be a Millionaire* and donated 10 percent of her winnings to 4-H, the nation's oldest youth development program where she is currently a member of the National Board of Trustees. She and her unique views have been featured on *E! True Hollywood Story*, NPR, PBS, *Inside Edition*, CBS's *The Early Show*, *Eyewitness Kids News*, Discovery Channel, *The Boston Globe*, *The Washington Post*, *USA Today*, *The New York Times*, *Forbes* magazine, ABC's *Good Morning America*, *CosmoGIRL!*, *J-14*, and more. She lives in Los Angeles.

## ANGELA DIAZ

Angela Diaz, M.D., M.P.H., is the director of the Mount Sinai Adolescent Health Center, the largest adolescent health center in the United States. Any teenager who comes through the Center's doors is provided the best care available—for free. Dr. Diaz is also president of The Children's Aid Society Board of Trustees, is a member of the FDA Pediatric Advisory Committee, and is a member of the New York City Board of Health.

Dr. Diaz has been a White House Fellow, and has been named numerous times as one of the Best Doctors in New York by *New York* magazine. Dr. Diaz has been providing direct medical services to children and adolescents for more than twenty-five years.